Blood Specimen Collection FAQs

answers to hundreds of the most frequently
asked questions on specimen collection

To purchase additional copies of this publication, call the Center for Phlebotomy Education's toll free number at 866-657-9857 or fax official purchase orders to 812-738-5750. Quantity discounts available.

Compiled by Dennis J. Ernst MT(ASCP).
Edited by Dennis J. Ernst MT(ASCP) & Lisa O. Ballance MT(ASCP).

Center for Phlebotomy Education, Inc.
P.O. Box 161
Ramsey, IN 47166
www.phlebotomy.com | phlebotomy@phlebotomy.com
Toll free phone: 866-657-9857

Every effort has been made to make this manual as complete and accurate as possible. The author and publisher have vigorously researched the information presented herein to be current with regard to product, product use, procedures, published articles and texts, and the national standards available and/or in effect at the time of publication. However, there may be errors both typographical and in content. Therefore, this document should be used only as a general guide and not as the ultimate source of blood specimen collection and processing information. Readers are advised to consult package inserts, current literature, legislation, and updated standards before applying the information contained herein.

The authors and publisher disclaim any and all responsibility for injury, loss, liability, or damage incurred directly or indirectly as a consequence of errors or omissions contained herein or of the implementation, application, and/or use of any of the information contained in this document. Neither the authors nor the publisher make any warranties, express or implied, to the contents of this publication.

Discussions on phlebotomy liability do not constitute legal advice. Neither the authors nor the publisher claim any responsibilty for the legal consequences resulting from the application of concepts discussed herein. Readers are advised to consult attorneys on any matters of legal liability.

Contents Overview

Contents

1. Safety & Infection Control

Safety

Contents

Contents

Certification

3. Skin Punctures, Heelsticks, & Pain Management

Skin Punctures/Heelsticks

Contents

Pain Management

Contents

4. Patient Identification, Vein Selection, & Site Prep

Patient Identification

Vein Selection

Contents

Site Prep

5. Tourniquets & Butterflies

Tourniquets

Contents

Butterflies

6. Order of Draw & Discard Tubes

Order of Draw

Discard Tubes

Contents

7. Hemolysis & Potassium Issues

Hemolysis

Potassium Issues

8. Blood Culture

Blood Culture

Contents

9. Labeling & Post-Venipuncture Care

Labeling

Post-Venipuncture Care

Contents

10. Line Draws & IV Starts

Line Draws & IV Starts

11. Processing, Storage, & Transportation

Processing

Contents

Storage & Transportation

12. Patient Injury & Complications

Patient Injury

Contents

Complications

13. Unorthodox Techniques

Unorthodox Techniques

Contents

14. Miscellaneous

Miscellaneous

Contents

Preface

It is the mission of the Center for Phlebotomy Education to be the most reliable source of information on blood specimen collection, to share that information in a variety of ways, and to elevate the status of the phlebotomy profession. For over 10 years, fulfilling that mission has meant answering tens of thousands of questions on blood specimen collection from healthcare professionals like you around the world.

Because many of the inquiries I receive are redundant of previously answered questions, the need for a published compendium of commonly asked questions and their answers has become obvious. You hold in your hands our response to that need.

To make this compilation more interesting than most FAQ collections, I've included the actual questions we've received from healthcare professionals around the world, not just a core question stripped of its context. Each one retains the human element that gives it life and dimension, and represents a multitude of similar inquiries on the same topic.

I've made it my job to keep current with what's published on the topic, and to contribute dozens of articles of my own. Because of my immersion in the subject, you can trust that the information contained in these pages is impeccably accurate and current with the prevailing standards and guidelines.

Ten years in the making, *Blood Specimen Collection FAQs* contains highly researched and referenced answers to the most commonly asked questions on phlebotomy. You should be able to find answers to your most burning questions in these pages. If not, ask me. I'll answer you by phone or email with an accurate, well-researched response.

It's what I do.

Respectfully,

Dennis J. Ernst MT(ASCP)
phlebotomy@phlebotomy.com
Toll free: 866-657-9857

1. Safety & Infection Control

Safety

Anchoring veins

Angle of insertion

Back-end needlestick injuries

Broken glass tubes

Contaminated tube holders

Ergonomics

Eye protection for venipunctures

Face shields and phlebotomy

Glass capillary tubes

Glove use and OSHA

Gloves during donor fingersticks

Lab coats

Letting blood drip from a needle hub

Letting blood drip from the IV cannula

OSHA and self-employed contractors

Plastic collection tubes

PPE for phlebotomy

Safety devices and two-handed activation

Staff resistant to glove use

Staff resistance to lab coats for phlebotomy

Infection Control

Anchoring veins

When we have new phlebotomists come through our lab for orientation, I'm finding several things wrong with their technique. One incident had to do with drawing in the "window" where the phlebotomist's index finger and thumb were above and below the venipuncture site, which made the rest of his hand at risk for a needlestick. However, the phlebotomy supervisor says the technique is okay.

Does CLSI address this specifically? I feel like I really need some absolutes to take to her and the lab manager. My goal is not to put anyone on the spot, but to train the staff according to the standards.

According to CLSI, the phlebotomist's thumb should be the only finger used to anchor the vein and stretch the skin, and that it should be one or two inches below the venipuncture site. Many textbooks also discourage using the two-finger technique in which the entry point of the vein is straddled by the index finger above and the thumb below. The risk is that the patient may jump or recoil upon needle insertion, and impale your index finger if it's in harm's way.

Angle of insertion

I've read and heard in many places that you should insert the needle at an angle of 30 degrees or less. How do you illustrate this to students? Do you bring a protractor along?

You are correct that most students wouldn't know what 30 degrees looks like. You might take a digital image of an approximation and put it in your materials or on a slide. In the absence of a visual, you can just state to enter the skin at the lowest angle possible. There is no minimum requirement to maintain, only the maximum. There are angle-of-insertion images to help you in the CLSI venipuncture standard. The standard can be obtained from the Clinical and Laboratory Standards Institute (www.clsi.org) or the Center for Phlebotomy Education (www.phlebotomy.com).

Back-end needlestick injuries

Prior to the Needlestick Safety and Prevention Act that became law in November 2001, how many cases are you aware of where a person was stuck with the back end of a needle, and do you have any details such as whether it happened when they removed the needle from the holder or not?

EPINet did a study on back-end needlesticks and published the results in Volume 6, Number 4 issue of *Advances in Exposure Prevention* (2003). According to the article, back-end needle injuries account for at least 10.5% of the needlesticks from phlebotomy needles (2000 & 2001 data).

The authors state the number may actually be higher. Unless the healthcare worker specifies in the description section of their report form which end of the needle caused the injury, it cannot be determined. The raw numbers are 12 of 114 reported injuries from phlebotomy needles in which the back end was specifically identified as the end that inflicted the puncture. In five of the twelve, needle removal was the mode of injury. The remaining seven accounts didn't specify the action involved.

Seven additional injuries were reported to have occurred while the needle was being removed, but the end that perforated the skin wasn't indicated in the description of the event, so they were not counted as confirmed back-end injuries. In actuality, the range could be as high as 17%. The statistics are based on between 50 to 70 hospitals reporting data to EPINet during that time.

Broken glass tubes

Please help settle a controversy in our laboratory. Our hospital uses a pneumatic tube system for specimen transport. Blood tubes are double-bagged in zip-lock biohazard bags for transport in the tube system. Recently, one of five blood tubes broke inside the bag. Some employees thought that all the tubes should be discarded and the patient re-collected. Others thought the intact tubes should be retrieved with tongs or forceps, cleaned, disinfected, and processed for testing. Is there a right or wrong answer here?

The immediate issue is whether or not to salvage intact tubes in a package that includes a broken tube and pooled blood. OSHA would probably insist on discarding the entire contaminated set rather than risk an exposure. It's a good bet that your infection control practitioner and risk manager would agree. Should a set of tubes be exposed to so much force during transportation that one tube breaks, there can be no guarantee that other tubes in the set are not cracked. Subsequent processing may result in a broken glass exposure during cleaning, handling, or centrifugation.

In our opinion, exposure prevention takes precedence over any patient priority. Should the laboratory establish a policy to the contrary, it opens itself up for liability should an employee suffer an exposure and acquire a pathogen.

The underlying issue the facility needs to address is its use of glass tubes. OSHA has made it quite clear in the Bloodborne Pathogens Standard, its Compliance Directives, and in statements from OSHA representatives that it expects facilities to convert to plastic tubes.[1-5] With the prevalence of plastic alternatives for all glass tubes, there is little justification for the continued use of glass.

(cont...)

(Broken glass tubes cont...)

References

1) US Department of Labor and Occupational Safety and Health Administration (OSHA). Occupational exposure to bloodborne pathogens; final rule (29 CFR 1910.1030). *Federal Register*.1991;Dec 6:64004–64182.

2) US Department of Labor and Occupational Safety and Health Administration (OSHA). Occupational exposure to bloodborne pathogens; final rule (29 CFR 1910.1030). http://www.osha.gov/pls/oshaweb/owadisp.show_document?p_table=STANDARDS&p_id=10051. Accessed 5/16/08.

3) US Department of Labor and Occupational Safety and Health Administration (OSHA). Enforcement Procedures for Occupational Exposure to Bloodborne Pathogens. CPL 2-2.69. http://www.osha.gov/pls/oshaweb/owadisp.show_document?p_table=DIRECTIVES&p_id=2570. Accessed 5/16/08.

4) Ernst D. Richard Fairfax of OSHA talks about the Bloodborne Pathogens Standard. *MLO* 2003;35(2):32–34.

5) Ernst D. Plastic Collection Tubes Decrease Risk of Employee Injury. *MLO* 2001;33(5):44–50.

Did You Know...

back problems alone cost American industry an estimated 16 billion dollars per year.

Contaminated tube holders

Q I am currently looking into the use of tube holders and supporting evidence on their contamination after one or multiple uses. Can you help?

A Several studies have been published on tube holder contamination. One showed a 9.2% visible contamination rate on tube holders.[1] A second study showed 48% were contaminated after one use (visible or invisible).[2] A third reported that 83% were positive for contamination with blood (visible or invisible).[3]

References

1) Howantiz P, Schifman R. Phlebotomists' safety practices. *Arch Pathol Lab Med* 1994;118:957-962.

2) Weinstein S, Hamrahi V, Popat A, Avato J, et al. Blood contamination of reusable needle holders. *Am J Inf Ctl* 1991;19(2).

3) Crawford D. Case Study: Phlebotomy. *Adv Admin Lab* 2000;9(1):70.

Ergonomics

One of our phlebotomists underwent knee surgery and told her manager that in order to work, she needed to sit on a stool. We all questioned the safety of this since it seems awkward to draw blood from a sitting position. An ergonomic study was done on this phlebotomist's behalf, and the report stated that all phlebotomists should be supplied with a stool. Am I right to question the validity of this as it relates to safety for both the phlebotomist and the patient?

The recommendation that came from the study is questionable. More ergonomic articles on phlebotomy concern back strain from bending over toward the patient than knee strain. That's why there's so much interest in ergonomic phlebotomy chairs and beds for patients, adjustable so that the patient can be brought up to the phlebotomist's level. Performing venipunctures from a sitting position could hamper the performance of the procedure. One needs to move more than what a sitting position would allow. It's understandable that a phlebotomist with a bad knee might need to keep her weight off it, but to prescribe stools for the entire staff seems to be an overreaction.

Eye protection for venipunctures

I have a question on proper eye protection for students in a phlebotomy program. Should phlebotomy students use a full-face shield, goggles, or safety glasses when performing venipunctures?

OSHA requires PPE when employers feel there is a risk of exposure. However, OSHA doesn't apply to students in an academic institution. So there is no legal mandate for eye protection when drawing blood in an academic setting. Since the risk of splashes to the eye during a routine venipuncture or skin puncture is very low, eyewear may not be necessary. It's up to the employer. You should contact the sites where you students will do their clinicals and see if they will require eyewear when your students arrive. If so, you should implement them in the classroom. However, the risk is significantly greater when your students remove stoppers and process specimens. If your students engage in this activity, you should require face protection.

Face shields and phlebotomy

I'm confused. Someone at a conference recently said face shields are required for phlebotomy. This is new to me and I want to make sure I'm not in violation of the standards. I'm afraid to call my local OSHA office for fear that they'll show up on my doorstep.

First of all, your fear is unfounded. OSHA actually wants to help you comply with the standards and would look favorably on your willingness to contact them for guidance.

The passage in the Bloodborne Pathogens Standard that addresses the issue reads as follows:

> *"Masks in combination with eye protection devices, such as goggles or glasses with solid side shields, or chin-length face shields, shall be worn whenever splashes, spray, spatter, or droplets of blood or other potentially infectious materials may be generated and eye, nose, or mouth contamination can be reasonably anticipated."*

Routine phlebotomy doesn't usually pose that risk, but it's up to the employer to make that determination. Some safety needles have a notice on their packages that warn against splatter. You might want to consider face protection when using these devices. However, if what you refer to as "routine phlebotomy" includes processing specimens, face protection is required since splashes are much more possible when stoppers are removed.

Glass capillary tubes

W e have been told to remove all glass microhematocrit tubes from our shelves and collection trays and outpatient drawing areas. However, we occasionally perform capillary blood gases in which a thick-walled, heparinized glass capillary tube is used. If we are to eliminate this device, how are we to perform capillary blood gases?

A s you may know, both OSHA and the CDC have mandated facilities eliminate the small, glass capillary tubes used for spun hematocrits. In fact, the use of glass microhematocrit tubes is an OSHA violation that can subject a facility to fines and citations. The manufacturing industry has responded to this ban by producing plastic or plastic-coated capillary tubes as a safer substitute. Plastic tubes for capillary blood gases are also available. One source is RAM Scientific (www.ramsci.com).

Glove use and OSHA

Our manager is writing us up for not wearing gloves when we draw blood. I've checked, and nowhere in the Bloodborne Pathogens Standard does it require gloves while drawing blood. Gloves do nothing to prevent the transmittance of any type of disease between patient and phlebotomist. She can't prove it. Can you?

Take a look at Section (d)(3)(ix) of the Bloodborne Pathogens Standard where it states:

"Gloves shall be worn... when performing vascular access procedures...."

There is also a passage in the OSHA document CPL 2–2.69, *Enforcement Procedures for Occupational Exposure to Bloodborne Pathogens*. (This document is the Compliance Directive, which instructs OSHA inspectors how to interpret and enforce the Standard. It's available on OSHA's web site to anyone with an interest in the Bloodborne Pathogens Standard.) In it, paragraph (d)(3)(ix) (A)–(C) reads:

"At a minimum, gloves must be used ...when performing vascular access procedures;"

It defines the one and only exception OSHA allows for employees not wearing gloves in Paragraph (d)(3)(ix)(D):

"The exemption regarding the use of gloves during phlebotomy procedures applies only to employees of volunteer donor blood collection centers, and does not apply to phlebotomy conducted in other settings such as plasmapheresis centers or hospitals."

Therefore, I think you'll agree OSHA is quite clear that gloves must be worn during venipuncture, the most common venous access procedure performed today.

As to your comment that "Wearing gloves while drawing blood does nothing to prevent the transmittance of any type of disease between patient and phlebotomist," I couldn't disagree more. It has been reported that there are over 20 different diseases that can be transmitted by blood contact. Again, from the Compliance Directive:

> *"Studies have shown that gloves provide a barrier, but that neither vinyl nor latex procedure gloves are completely impermeable."*

Gloves are not impermeable, but here's a hypothetical to think about: Let's say you have a break in the skin on your fingertip and you are in the middle of drawing a patient with hepatitis or HIV. The patient suddenly jerks, causing the needle to come out of his vein, and blood to pool on his skin. Are you going to stop and put your gloves on before reaching for the gauze and applying pressure? No, you're going to release the tourniquet, reach for the gauze and stop the bleeding. The blood that pools on his skin while you collect your thoughts will saturate the gauze quickly and make contact with the broken skin on your finger.

There's more. Studies show that when a contaminated needle pierces a glove, the material of the glove serves to wipe off up to 86 percent of the blood volume the needle will deliver into your skin.[1] That means you have a lesser inoculation of whatever virus could be in the blood that infects you.

Remember, your patients and your family need you to continue being there for them. Take care of yourself so you can.

Reference

1) Mast S, Woolwine J, Gerberding J. Efficacy of gloves in reducing blood volumes transferred during simulated needlestick injury. *J Infect Dis* 1993;168(6):1589–1592.

Gloves during donor fingersticks

I went to a blood drive at our church recently and the phlebotomist didn't wear gloves when she was doing my fingerstick hemoglobin check. She said she wasn't required to, but would if I asked her to. I did, of course, because she wasn't even washing hands between patients. I called the head of the blood center on Monday and he said OSHA told him gloves do not have to be worn because we are not patients, but donors. Is this true?

Yes. Here's what OSHA says in its Bloodborne Pathogens Standard about wearing gloves in blood donor centers:

> *"If an employer in a volunteer blood donation center judges that routine gloving for all phlebotomies is not necessary, then the employer shall...periodically reevaluate this policy; make gloves available to all employees who wish to use them for phlebotomy; not discourage the use of gloves for phlebotomy; and require that gloves be used for phlebotomy in the following circumstances: when the employee has cuts, scratches, or other breaks in his or her skin; when the employee judges that hand contamination with blood may occur, for example, when performing phlebotomy on an uncooperative source individual; and when the employee is receiving training in phlebotomy."*

OSHA leaves it up to the employee to judge the risk. Here is what the Standard says about handwashing:

Section 1910.1030(d)(2)(vi): *"Employers shall ensure that employees wash hands and any other skin with soap and water, or flush mucous membranes with water immediately or as soon as feasible following contact of such body areas with blood or other potentially infectious materials."*

According to this passage, the hands would have to be contaminated with blood in order for handwashing to be required. Although not required, blood donor centers would be well advised to instruct screeners to cleanse hands between donors, at least as a matter of infection control, hygiene, and customer service.

Did You Know...

eight to seventeen percent of healthcare workers are at risk for adverse reactions from exposure to latex.

Lab coats

I work as a safety officer in an independent lab. Our phlebotomists work in draw stations and wear lab coats when they draw blood. The hospital phlebotomists wear scrubs, which are not removed before leaving the premises or before going to lunch. Likewise, nurses also wear the same clothing home and around the hospital. We don't have standards or experts that say that the hospital should take on the expense of lab coats as personal protective equipment (PPE) and their laundering. To me it is common sense for infection control purposes. What's the bottom line on wearing and laundering lab coats?

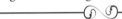

Your situation is typical of many facilities, i.e., phlebotomists wear scrubs without protective lab coats. OSHA consultants will tell you that wearing lab coats over scrubs is not necessary if phlebotomists only perform venipunctures and skin punctures. But if phlebotomists also process specimens (e.g., remove stoppers, transfer serum, rim clots, clean blood spills, etc.), PPE is required by OSHA's Bloodborne Pathogens Standard as a circumstance in which exposure can be reasonably anticipated.

In this case, that would be face protection, gloves and impermeable lab coats. In addition, the standard states that it is the employer's responsibility to launder lab coats if their use is mandated.

Letting blood drip from a needle hub

Do you have any information on a phlebotomy procedure called "drip" or "free flow"? My understanding is that this is a procedure for collecting blood specimens on babies. A small gauge needle is inserted in a vein on the top of the baby's hand, and blood is allowed to drip out the hub of the needle into a micro-collection tube.

This technique does not appear in the literature and should be discouraged as a homespun modification. The risk of a bloodborne pathogen exposure is obvious. You don't see this procedure described in the textbooks for a reason.

Letting blood drip from the IV cannula

To avoid an extra stick, our nurses use the patients' IV sites for blood collection before hooking up fluids or meds. They do not attach a syringe though, but merely allow the blood to drip into the collection tube (red- and purple-tops only). Syringes were used at first, but hemolysis and clotting became a problem. Is there anything wrong with this method of collection? Can you provide any sort of written protocol or procedure for this?

Your description of letting the blood trickle into the tube is chilling. Such a technique is rather contrived and risks exposure. You won't find this technique in any textbook or standard, as it is an unconventional approach and fraught with risk.

The hemolysis they experienced is inherent when drawing blood through an IV. Such devices simply aren't meant to be used for that purpose, and are notorious for hemolyzing specimens. (Up to ten times more likely according to some studies.) Sometimes you can get away with it, but other times, a venipuncture has to be performed when the specimen gets rejected for hemolysis.

I suspect the clotting problem experienced in the past is a result of setting down the blood-filled syringe and tending to the IV fluids. Meanwhile, the blood clots in the syringe. When drawing blood during an IV start or from an existing IV device, an assistant is necessary so the specimen can be transferred to the tubes immediately. You should try to discourage draws during IV starts where possible. They're nothing but a headache. You should also squelch the practice of letting blood drip into the tube.

OSHA and self-employed contractors

I am a paramedical examiner. While the company provides me with a safety needle and tube holder for each patient, I am instructed *not* to put the tube holders in the sharps container. I am to unscrew the safety needle, drop it into the sharps container, then dispose of the used tube holder in the regular garbage. I feel this is contradictory and unsafe. Can I use one of those auto-release tube holders that drop the needle into the sharps container with the click of a button? The problem is that I am a contractor and not an employee, so technically I cannot "demand" safer work accommodations.

Don't be so sure you can't demand safer work accommodations. Whether or not your employer is obligated to maintain safe work practices for you depends on the terms of your contract. If your terms indicate that you have an employer-employee relationship, then they would have to supply you with equipment and devices that are OSHA-compliant. They would also have to be responsible for your hepatitis immunizations, post-exposure management, Bloodborne Pathogens training, and all the other provisions of the Bloodborne Pathogens Standard. But if your contract indicates that you do not have an employee relationship, and that you work independently, which is what you seemed to indicate is the case, then they would not be subject to OSHA standards as they apply to work you do on their behalf. But the terms of your agreement might be written in such a way that they still have some employer responsibilities. It's going to ultimately be up to an OSHA inspector to determine.

As an indicator, It seems that since they're providing you with your immunizations, they're taking on the responsibilities of an employer for a reason. Perhaps it's worded in your contract that they serve in that capacity.

The sticky part is that OSHA cannot cite an employer who cannot monitor compliance, such as whether a visiting nurse uses gloves during vascular access procedures in the home or not. Or if a paramedical examiner activates a safety device in the applicant's home. But if you are an employee and your employer

(cont...)

cannot monitor compliance, they're not likely to be exempt from putting OSHA-compliant devices in your hands. Providing them is one thing; making sure you activate the safety feature when you are in patients' homes is another.

If you do have an employee-employer arrangement, their insistence that you remove the needle and dispose of them separately is a violation of OSHA standards. The employer can be fined and issued a citation for making you perform in this manner.

Since they are instructing you to do so, a dual relationship suddenly exists that might qualify the company you contract with as a "controlling employer." Because there are so many conditions and variables involved in your case, you should consult with your state's/region's OSHA office for clarification. They're good at sorting these things out. If it turns out that the company is not bound to OSHA guidelines, then it's up to you to take the necessary steps to protect yourself. That would mean buying your own sharps containers. The auto-release devices you mentioned are not OSHA-compliant, but they're safer than removing the needle by hand.

You should think twice about working for a contractor who insists you engage in hazardous practices... like removing needles from tube holders. Insist on having the equipment necessary to protect yourself from accidental needlesticks. If they tell you to take a hike, so be it. They can probably find someone desperate enough to compromise their own safety to replace you, but at least your health and well-being won't be at risk.

Plastic collection tubes

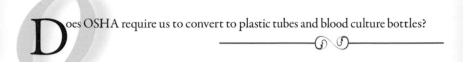

Does OSHA require us to convert to plastic tubes and blood culture bottles?

Here's what an OSHA representative had to say on the issue:
"*The first line of safety in the industrial hygiene hierarchy is substitution. If there is a plastic substitute for glass, it should be implemented. Whether it's citation worthy would depend on the circumstances of the case, use of the glass, work practices, contamination, etc., etc. And, glass contaminated with blood or other potentially infectious materials(OPIM) must always be placed in a sharps container (one that is puncture resistant, leakproof, and closable), regardless of whether it's broken or not, just like all other sharps. The key here is prevention. Preventing the glass from breaking saves so many more potential exposures downstream.*" OSHA leaves it up to the employer to judge the risk.

There are plenty of passages in OSHA documents and statements from OSHA authorities that also shed light on how the agency feels about converting from glass to plastic in the laboratory. Consider the following passage from Section (d)(2)(i) in the Standard:[1]

"*engineering and work practice controls shall be used to eliminate or minimize employee exposure.*"

The latest Compliance Directive instructs inspectors how to interpret this passage:[2]

"*Where engineering controls will reduce employee exposure either by removing, eliminating, or isolating the hazard, they must be used.*"

(cont...)

(Plastic collection tubes cont...)

Most managers think of this passage in terms of safety needles and stop there. Even though this passage remains unchanged from the original standard, OSHA modified its definition of "engineering controls" in 2001 in such a way so as to include other equipment. Changes to the original document have been italicized.

Original definition: Engineering controls: "controls (e.g., sharps disposal containers, self-sheathing needles) that isolate or remove the bloodborne pathogens hazard from the workplace."

Revised definition: Engineering controls: "controls (e.g., sharps disposal containers, self-sheathing needles, *safer medical devices, such as sharps with engineered sharps injury protection and needleless systems*) that isolate or remove the bloodborne pathogens hazard from the workplace."

The inclusion of "safer medical devices" in the revised definition reflects OSHA's intent to broaden the definition to cover other devices, sharps with engineered sharps injury protection being only one example.

A passage in Section (d)(2)(i) of the latest Compliance Directive provides further evidence that the use of glass blood collection tubes subjects the employer to OSHA citation and fines.

"If no engineering controls are being used to eliminate or minimize exposure, a citation should be issued."

Then there are these statements by Richard Fairfax, OSHA's Director of Enforcement Programs, in an interview published in *MLO* magazine:

"Since plastic can be easily substituted for glass in most all cases, we expect employers to use plastic where appropriate.... Since plastic tubes are readily available that do not compromise specific clinical or diagnostic tests, a facility that is not using them would have to justify why they are not being used for each specific procedure or test, and document that in their exposure control plan."

But eliminating as much glass in your facilities as possible is not just to satisfy OSHA. Statistics based on EPINet data show an average of 4924 healthcare workers suffer broken glass exposures each year from blood specimen collection tubes.[3]

References

1) US Department of Labor and Occupational Safety and Health Administration (OSHA). Occupational exposure to bloodborne pathogens; final rule (29 CFR 1910.1030). *Federal Register*.1991;Dec 6:64004–64182.

2) OSHA Compliance Directive 2-2.69. Available: http://www.osha.gov/pls/oshaweb/owadisp.show_document?p_table=DIRECTIVES&p_id=2570. Accessed 5/16/08.

3) Exposure Prevention Information Network (EPINet) Data Reports. International Health Care Worker Safety Center, University of Virginia. 2000."Available at http://www.healthsystem.virginia.edu/internet/epinet/EPINet-2003-report.pdf. Accessed 5/16/08.

Did You Know...

two out of five nurses surveyed wouldn't recommend their health care facility to a family member.

PPE for phlebotomy

We have been having a discussion as to what is required PPE when performing phlebotomy. Where can I find the requirements?

Gloves are required by OSHA when performing phlebotomy. Lab coats and face protection are required when removing stoppers during processing. Foot protection when processing specimens should include shoes that do not expose toes, heels or any other part of the foot. They should be easily cleaned if a spill occurs.

Generally, OSHA requires personal protective equipment whenever exposure can be reasonably anticipated. Much of this is dependent upon what the employer considers "reasonably anticipated." However, glove use is one PPE that is mandated in the Bloodborne Pathogens Standard when drawing blood specimens, either by fingerstick or venipuncture.

For much longer articles on this subject than can be printed here, consider volume 1 of the *To the Point*™ series of CEU exercises subtitled "Collection Protection." It is available at www.phlebotomy.com.

Safety devices and two-handed activation

Our organization was recently told by a vendor that safety devices on phlebotomy products should be activated single handedly. After much research, I haven't been able to find a reference to this. Was this vendor pulling my leg?

There's no leg-pulling going on here. The vendor is referring to a publication put out by the National Institute for Occupational Safety and Health (NIOSH).[1] It states:

"A number of sources have identified the desirable characteristics of safety devices. The characteristics include the following..."

It goes on to list eight characteristics; one of them is that the "safety feature can be engaged with a single-handed technique." Note that these are recommended safety features, not OSHA mandates. However, according to OSHA, if safer devices are available, they must be used. Therefore, it's conceivable that an inspector could come in, find that you are using safety devices that require two hands to activate, and cite you because devices that require one hand to activate are available, but not being used. You might avoid a citation in this situation if your exposure control plan shows that you tried the "safer" device and found that it was less effective than the two-handed device currently in use. It's hard to believe that to be possible, though, and might be a tough sell to an inspector.

Reference

1) National Institute for Occupational Safety and Health (NIOSH). *Preventing Needlestick Injuries in Health Care Settings*, Free publication from NIOSH, Publications Dissemination, 4676 Columbia Parkway, Cincinnati, OH 45226. 800-356-4674 or download from www.cdc.gov/niosh.

Staff resistant to glove use

Do you have any resources that address the issue of staff not wearing gloves to draw blood? I work in a nice suburban hospital and this is a big issue. They just do not want to wear gloves.

What you described is unfortunate, but not uncommon. There are at least three major documents that your staff is challenging:

1.) The OSHA Bloodborne Pathogens Standard;

2.) your facility policy, which should reflect the OSHA standard;

3.) CLSI standard H3-A6. *Procedures for the Collection of Diagnostic Blood Specimens by Venipuncture.*

Nothing else matters. Wearing gloves is one of those things that everyone knows, so there really is no excuse. Those who don't wear gloves make a conscious choice to violate facility policy and, by so doing, subject the facility to OSHA fines and citations. Issuing a facility-wide warning is in order, telling the staff that the policy will be enforced consistently in the future. Then, spell out what the consequences will be for employees caught performing vascular access procedures without gloves.

Some people need to be protected from themselves. They don't stop to realize their cavalier approach is putting them and everyone who loves and relies on them at risk of losing them to preventable hepatitis, HIV, etc. The facility has a moral and legal obligation to enforce glove use for all vascular access procedures. Don't take any whining from your staff about being unable to perform the procedure. Millions of healthcare workers have adapted; they can, too.

Stuck with a clean needle

What should we do if we stick ourselves with a *clean* needle?

Check with your infection control department on how your facility wants you to react to wounds inflicted by clean needles. There's nothing in the standards that shed much light on this issue. I would suggest the wound be washed to prevent contamination from skin bacteria and cover the site to prevent contamination while you work. Hepatitis B lives on surfaces for up to a week, so make sure you don't expose yourself to potentially contaminated surfaces. If the clean needlestick is severe, you might want to be treated in your ED, but much of this is dependent upon your facility's policy.

Syringe draw safety

A phlebotomist drew blood from a patient in a syringe, and then stuck the syringe needle into the tube stopper to let the vacuum pull the blood into the tube. Several other phlebotomists said this was not an acceptable practice. They say the sample would be hemolyzed and/or clot in the syringe. Are they right?

Your phlebotomists are right, but for the wrong reason. It's best that blood does not impact the bottom of the tube full force, but rather flows down the side of the tube to prevent hemolysis. But, this is secondary to a much larger issue.

Piercing the stopper of the tube with the same needle that was used to draw the blood is not safe and violates OSHA regulations. The risk of the needle accidentally piercing the finger is too great. The proper procedure for filling tubes from a syringe is to activate the safety needle after the needle is removed from the vein, remove it from the syringe, discard it immediately, apply a safety transfer device, and fill the tubes.

A safety transfer device is like a tube holder that threads onto the syringe, and has an interior needle to fill the tubes, just like with a tube-holder draw. They're widely available. Clotting in the barrel of the syringe is only an issue if the draw takes a long time, and the blood sits in the syringe for a prolonged period.

Syringes versus tube holders and butterflies

I am originally from New York City where phlebotomists are provided with as many butterfly needles as we desire. I moved to East Texas recently where they dole out only a few butterflies per month. Instead, they have us use syringes. We then have to change the needle and transfer into tubes! I think this is crazy... maybe illegal. A girl who just arrived from Connecticut has the same story. Please advise me about this situation! I'm desperate. I am even willing to purchase my own butterflies.

Butterfly needles have been associated with a high rate of accidental needlesticks.[1] They are expensive and often overused. Even though your comfort zone is built around butterfly use, it's not generally in your best interest to use them exclusively.

Removing the needle from syringes and applying a safety transfer device to fill the tubes isn't illegal. In fact, it's the method OSHA prefers you use when drawing into a syringe, provided you are using a safety needle and activating the feature first.

Syringes are the device most healthcare workers use when they suffer an accidental needlestick. Their use is discouraged in most of the literature and in the CLSI standards. But some situations call for a syringe. Like butterfly sets, they should be used only when the situation calls for them.

Try to use a tube holder with a multi-sample needle whenever you think the vein can withstand the constant pressure of the vacuum tube when it is pushed onto the interior needle. Tube holders attached to needles are easier, less expensive, safer, and more convenient.

Reference

1) Jagger J. (1994) Risky procedure, risky devices, risky job. *Adv Exp Prev* 1994;1(1):4–9.

Tube holder reuse

I am a patient who recently had my blood collected. I noticed a speck of blood on the plastic tube holder near the threaded area. The phlebotomist assured me that I had nothing to worry about, since it is common to reuse this plastic piece, and that this part does not touch the patient or the sterile needle. Nevertheless, I'm concerned that I might have been exposed to someone else's blood. Should I be worried?

The use of a dirty tube holder during your venipuncture is unacceptable on many levels. However, the risk of transmission of bloodborne diseases is negligible.

The phlebotomist is correct that the needle attached to the tube holder through the contaminated threads does not come in contact with the patient. Nevertheless, he/she is misinformed that the tube holder can be reused. It has been very highly publicized that OSHA does not allow the tube holders to be reused. They are to be thrown away after one use.

You can pursue this in several ways. Contact the laboratory manager and see what the official policy is at the facility. Perhaps the phlebotomist was acting against the employer's policy and simply needs to be corrected. If the lab manager states that reusing tube holders is appropriate, then the facility is not operating within the OSHA standard. I would find another facility for your future blood work.

When to glove

The current approved standard for venipuncture indicates you should put gloves on before you cleanse the site. I teach my students to cleanse first, then glove so that the site can dry while they put on their gloves. Too often I see phlebotomists cleanse the site, and then rub it dry so that they can proceed with the venipuncture. If they had something to do while the alcohol dries, like put on gloves, they wouldn't be wiping off the alcohol, but letting it dry like they should. Could it be acceptable to cleanse the site before putting on gloves?

You are correct about the CLSI order of gloving and cleansing, and you have a valid point. It could be argued either way.

To the patient, it may be more welcome if the hands that cleanse their arm are gloved so that they feel they are less likely to be on the receiving end of an infection. Not that they would be more susceptible, but the perception to the patient is that infection control has a higher priority when put on prior to cleansing.

There are plenty of other things your students can do while waiting for the alcohol to dry, like assemble the needle, gather the tubes, organize the supplies, etc. Being a volatile substance, alcohol only takes a few seconds to dry, so rushing to get on with the procedure by wiping off the alcohol is simply nervous energy at work. Remind them that alcohol kills some bacteria if it's allowed to dry. Maybe that's all they need to know.

When to remove gloves

Our facility's self-inspection teams have dinged our staff for removing gloves before labeling blood specimens. Are they being too picky? What would you consider safe practice?

When the gloves come off is pretty much up to the employer, but you have to consider that OSHA insists gloves be worn "during vascular access procedures." Keep in mind that the agency's Bloodborne Pathogens Standard from which this passage comes doesn't define when the "procedure" officially ends. But it's obvious why you would want the staff to consider labeling as part of the venipuncture procedure.

Setting that argument aside, OSHA also states that employers must mandate personal protective equipment (such as gloves) when exposure can be "reasonably anticipated." If your staff is labeling tubes before the puncture site is bandaged, exposure can be reasonably anticipated during the bandaging process, especially if the patient continues to bleed after pressure is applied. In this case, you would be justified to mandate that gloves remain in place until the patient is bandaged. If your staff is labeling tubes after bandaging is complete, removing the gloves before labeling may pose a less risk of exposure. But you would still have to wrestle with the OSHA mandate that gloves be worn during the procedure, and that the procedure is not complete until the specimen is labeled.

One is hard-pressed to find a valid reason to remove gloves prior to labeling. The practice is probably just a matter of comfort. Those who are "dinging" your staff for early glove removal are interpreting the OSHA standard literally, and have the stronger argument.

"Windows" technique

I have a phlebotomy extern doing clinicals at my facility. Her instructor is teaching that it is "illegal" to anchor veins by putting the index finger above the site and the thumb below the site, then stretching to anchor.

Our phlebotomists use this method routinely, saying it anchors better and minimizes the discomfort for patients. It seems that the only risk of being stuck is going in, with a clean needle. When the needle is likely to come out, the phleb is no longer anchoring. Can you think of any reason this should be discouraged?

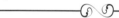

This technique, also called creating a "window," is dangerous and should be discouraged.

Here's a hypothetical for your staff to consider: what if the patient jumps upon needle insertion? More than likely, the needle comes out of the patient's flesh and goes immediately into the phlebotomist's finger, precariously positioned above the puncture site. Or, what if someone bumps the phlebotomist from behind at the time of greatest vulnerability? These things happen, and when they do, those who put themselves at risk are plunged into six months of waiting, testing, and sheer anxiety until they know for sure they haven't acquired hepatitis, HIV or any of the other 20 diseases known to be transmitted by blood exposure.

Many veteran phlebotomists use this technique, but it's to their own peril.

Artificial fingernails

The matter of fake nails has been an issue at our company for some time now. My employer has made it policy that no fake nails or overlays are to be worn if you are involved with patient care, even though we are wearing gloves. I would like to know what you think would be better: a nice manicure that is being taken care of, or stubby, bleeding skin, torn from constant biting?

Tidy fingernails are important from an infection control standpoint. Of course, poor nail care and bleeding cuticles are as much of a hazard as long, flashy extensions. Policies should ban both. According to a recently revised hand-hygiene guideline issued by the CDC's Healthcare Infection Control Practices Advisory Committee, there should be no artificial nails or extenders in the ICU or OR.[1,2]

The report states that, although the contribution of artificial nails to the transmission of infections is not known, healthcare workers who wear artificial nails are more likely to harbor gram-negative pathogens on the fingertips both before and after hand washing than those who have natural nails. It also reports that the majority of bacterial growth on the nail occurs within 1 mm of the skin. Personnel wearing artificial nails have been implicated in outbreaks of bacterial and yeast infections.

According to the "Hand Hygiene Guideline Factsheet" posted on the CDC web site, "Health care personnel should avoid wearing artificial nails and keep natural nails less than one quarter of an inch long if they care for patients at high risk of acquiring infections."[3]

Because nosocomial infections have been estimated to cause 100,000 deaths in the US each year (20,000 from poor hand hygiene alone), it's a serious problem that requires policies as strict as what your employer has established.[4] Although I'm sure you are keeping your nails nicely groomed, there's too much evidence against artificial nails of any length for an argument. Nicely groomed artificial nails may be better than chapped, bleeding cuticles, but they are still hazardous to the patient.

References

1) Bjerke N. Hand hygiene in healthcare: playing by the new rules. *Inf Ctl Today* Feb, 2003. 49–51.

2) Boyce J, Pittet D. Guideline for hand hygiene in healthcare settings: recommendations of the Healthcare Infection Control Practices Advisory Committee and the PICPAC/SHEA/APIC Hand Hygiene Task Force. *MMWR* October 25,2002.51(RR16);1–44.

3) CDC. Hand Hygiene Guideline Factsheet. http://www.cdc.gov/od/oc/media/pressrel/fs021025.htm. Accessed 5/16/08.

4) Berens, M. Tribune investigation: unhealthy hospitals. *Chicago Tribune*. July 21, 2002. http://www.ahrp.org/infomail/0702/23.php. Accessed 5/16/08.

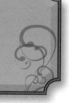

Did You Know...

one hospital estimated the cost of an acquired latex allergy to an employee to be over $157,000 over five years.

Discarding tourniquets

Has OSHA ruled that tourniquets in the outpatient setting must be discarded after each patient, or only when soiled or at the end of day? I am looking for the actual regulation, not opinion.

OSHA would not make such a mandate. Discarding tourniquets after one use is more of an infection control issue than an OSHA issue. OSHA is concerned only with employee injury and illness, not patient matters. In fact, OSHA doesn't even mention tourniquets in the Bloodborne Pathogens Standard, so the agency has no position on the subject unless the equipment is soiled by blood in such a manner and to such a degree that it is a potential risk to employees.

What OSHA does say is this: "All equipment and environmental and working surfaces shall be cleaned and decontaminated after contact with blood or other potentially infectious materials.... Special care shall be taken to avoid skin contact with other potentially infectious materials."

So it's really up to your facility to establish the policy based on current infection control policies and this OSHA passage. It's generally accepted that tourniquets be discarded when visibly soiled. Your infection control officer should be consulted and a policy should be drafted based on his/her recommendations. Establishing a policy that visibly soiled tourniquets be discarded should be the bare minimum. Facilities vary widely in their policies on tourniquet disposal. I'm seeing more and more of them are adopting a single-use policy to fight nosocomial infections, and would encourage you to consider one as well.

Keep in mind, over 75,000 patients die every year from preventable nosocomial infections. It's hard to believe that contaminated tourniquets don't contribute to the problem.

Reusing needles

It's my understanding that the American Diabetes Association considers it acceptable for diabetics to reuse their own insulin syringes. That indicates to me that it's okay to use the same needle for multiple punctures on the same patient. So if I miss the vein, I can take the needle out and reuse it on the same patient during the same draw, right?

That logic doesn't work. There's a fundamental difference between a patient using the same needle on him/herself and a healthcare professional reusing a needle on the same patient.

The American Diabetes Association does not set the standard for blood collection procedures, nor should they be considered an authoritative source of specimen collection information. Applying their rationale for your work on patients is applying things out of context. I think the ADA would agree.

There are many reasons why a needle used for phlebotomy should not be reused:

1.) Each time you pierce the tissue and remove the needle from the skin, tissue fluid accumulates inside. Puncture after unsuccessful puncture, it can potentially contaminate the specimen and alter test results once the vein is accessed and the fluid taken into the sample. Once the needle is removed from the skin, it should be considered "dirty," inside and out. The accumulation of tissue fluid and skin cells may not be a problem when diabetics give themselves insulin, but is a problem when drawing blood.

2.) From a patient's standpoint, it can be disturbing to see the same needle being used on multiple attempts. It's a customer service issue, and the practice of starting completely over with a new needle gives the patient confidence in the healthcare professional's respect for sterility.

(cont...)

(Reusing needles cont...)

3.) If the vein is missed and the needle is withdrawn and reinserted into another area, chances are you will palpate for the vein again, and again contaminating the site. Once cleansed, a puncture site should never be repalpated. The glove is not sterile, and cleansing the tip of the glove is not considered an acceptable alternative.

4.) If the vein is missed and the needle removed, you may be tempted to set it aside so that another site can be palpated and cleansed. This violates OSHA's Bloodborne Pathogens Standard, which states that contaminated needles must be immediately discarded into a sharps container. If the used needle is resheathed while an alternative site or vein is located, this is also a clear and serious violation of OSHA standards, which states that needles must not be recapped.

I hope this convinces you not to apply the American Diabetes Association's recommendations for diabetics to your technique in drawing blood specimens.

Did You Know...

3% of the anesthesiologists who responded to a survey said they reuse needles and/or syringes on multiple patients. (source: healthsafetyinfo.com)

Sterile versus non-sterile gauze

Since the recent media craze surrounding MRSA, an interesting issue came to my attention as a phlebotomy supervisor of a community hospital. An outpatient at our draw station was shocked to see that we do not use "sterile" gauze when drawing his blood. He became so irate that he demanded to be directed to the CEO. We have always used 2x2 gauze sponges packaged in a small 200-sponge "non-sterile" pack for use with venipuncture. I am afraid I will be hearing from our CEO, and I want to assure them that we follow the most current standards with our phlebotomy practice. Should we be using sterile, single-packaged gauze pads?

Phlebotomy is not considered a sterile procedure. According to the CLSI venipuncture standard, "clean" gauze is sufficient. It's also in line with what most facilities use. So you are consistent with the standards and the norm. That said, your facility may opt to go one better and use sterile gauze to placate your patients.

If/when your CEO addresses this issue with you, explain that you are in keeping with the standards. The risk of inducing an infection only because the "clean" gauze is not sterile is infinitesimal. Explain also that nurses more than likely don't use sterile gauze when giving injections, flushing ports, performing TB skin tests, etc. So I'm of the opinion that if your CEO wants to implement sterile gauze for venipuncture, you should be prepared to make it facility-wide.

But there is an opportunity here to have a significant impact in your facility on a much higher level. A far greater risk for nosocomial infections is the common practice of using the same tourniquet on multiple patients. This might be a good opportunity for you to bring about a change in several infection control policies. Think of the sweeping changes you could facilitate that could significantly reduce your facility's nosocomial infection rate. Bring your infection control person in on the conversation and take advantage of this opportunity.

Where to set phlebotomy trays

Regarding infection control, our phlebotomists want to know the safest place to set their phlebotomy tray in a patient's room. The floor seems unacceptable, the bedside table is occupied with personal effects, the eating table seems inappropriate as does the bed, and the chair is usually occupied with personal effects. We do use carts for morning draws, but use trays for efficiency the remainder of the day. What's the recommendation?

You should avoid patient surfaces (night stand, bedside table, bed) at all costs. Instead, have them place their phlebotomy trays on a surface neither the patient nor the patient's personal items are likely to become directly exposed to, such as a chair. Avoid the temptation to place the tray directly on the patient's bed since it may be inadvertently kicked onto the floor by sudden movements. You might also consider routinely cleansing the bottom and sides of your trays with a solution of 10% bleach.

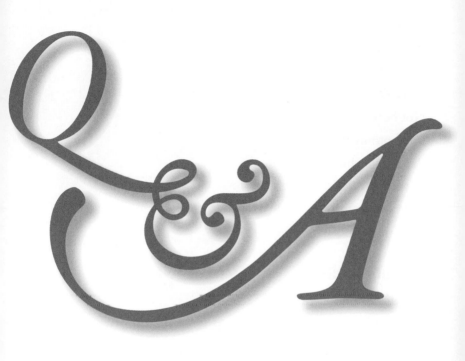

2. Training, Management, & Certification

Training

Learning phlebotomy in eight hours

Minimum in-house training

Nervous student

Not born to teach

Phlebotomy training

Reputable phlebotomy schools

Student clinicals

Switching hands

Teaching hand-switching

Management

Decentralized phlebotomy

Decentralized phlebotomy & failed venipuncture attempts

Decentralized phlebotomy stats

Disciplining phlebotomists

Draws per hour

Interviewing new phlebotomists

Maintaining competency

Minimum age for phlebotomists

Motivating phlebs

Certification

Learning phlebotomy in eight hours

My sister is an LPN and she told me that I can take an eight-hour class to become a phlebotomist. I would like very much to become a phlebotomist, so if you can help me find such a course, it would be most appreciated.

Becoming a phlebotomist takes more than eight hours. You might be able to learn the basics, but actually becoming a phlebotomist takes much more. I wouldn't spend your money on a phlebotomy course with that expectation unless it was at least 50 hours long, and includes drawing from actual patients. There are schools that will teach it in eight hours, but don't expect any employer to recognize it as proper training. For a list of schools in your area, visit www.phlebotomy.com and click on "School Directories."

Minimum in-house training

Q I am an MT teaching a hospital phlebotomy class for nurses and patient service assistants. I am curious on the length of training at other facilities. What is the recommended curriculum and time to completion?

A There really is no recommended time of training outside of California, which mandates 80 classroom hours plus 50 supervised punctures and completion of a certification exam. Start with that as a benchmark. Getting your administrator(s) to grant you that many hours may be a challenge, but seek approval for as many hours as you can get. Most facilities struggle with getting other departments to understand why so much time is necessary. If you can get even 20 classroom hours, you're doing better than most. Shoot for 50 supervised punctures and successful completion of a written and practical exam.

Press for making it mandatory that nurses who draw blood spend a day rotating through the lab to see what happens to specimens. Even half a day would be better than none.

Nervous student

I currently have a student who I am training to draw blood. She shakes terribly and hesitates to put the needle under the skin. I have tried many things to get her over this, but she still hesitates every time she is close to inserting the needle. I have done one-on-one with no other students around; I've asked her to bring a friend who she would not be nervous with; I've tried having someone she does not know to draw; I've talked, distracted, and tried other psychological approaches. Nothing is working and I'm out of options. She's fine with the phlebotomy arm, but not real flesh. Any suggestions?

I'll assume your student shakes because she's nervous, not because she has any condition. If it's nervousness and you've exhausted all other options, it may be time for extremes in order to salvage this student.

First, consider hypnosis. If she's fine with needles on artificial arms, but not on live flesh, there might be some deeply suppressed fear that has gone unresolved. Hypnosis has proven to be very successful in getting people past their fears.

Secondly, consider that perhaps the leap from artificial to real is too great, and she needs an incremental step that can serve as a bridge. Try taking her hand in yours and guiding the needle into a volunteer's arm for her. Let her hold the needle, but let your hand guide hers while advancing it into the vein. Once in the flesh, immediately remove the needle and bandage the volunteer. Don't even worry about putting tubes on or getting blood.

On the next attempt, you could provide a little less of the advancement pressure and so on until she is advancing the needle herself with your hand still in place on hers. Eventually, you can add additional steps to the procedure such as filling one tube, then multiple tubes, etc. Then gradually reduce your assistance.

There's another way to provide an intermediate step that will transition her from drawing on an artificial training arm to a live draw. Is it possible for you to arrange for her to practice on a cadaver? Sure, it's extreme, but perhaps it's the bridge she needs.

Not born to teach

I feel I am a knowledgeable phlebotomist, and I can quickly tell if a person has or will develop the skill to become a well-trained phlebotomist. Yet I lack the patience to teach. Our facility gets numerous students, but I cringe at the thought of training them. Can you give me some hints on how to become more patient with students who don't catch on quickly?

It's very easy for people to get impatient with those who don't have the passion we do for good technique or the willingness to learn. Everyone is different and unique in their own way, and everyone has something special that they bring to their job. It helps for trainers to keep in mind that they themselves were once incompetent and lacked the skills they now have. For every successful trainer, there's someone who once invested in them their patience.

The challenge for you is to reinvest that patience in others, even if it seems they are beyond hope. It's all about "grooming" people to develop into caring, compassionate, skillful phlebotomists.

People will either take to phlebotomy or they won't. But very few take to it instantly. When exposed to the proper environment long enough, a grain of sand eventually becomes a beautiful pearl. The challenge for trainers is to see the potential for a pearl in every grain of sand, and provide the environment... even when it drives them bonkers. It's all about patience.

Keep in mind, not everyone is wired to teach, either. If you are certain that you are one of them, then it's good to realize it and accept your limitations. Only you can make that decision. But give it some time and deep thought. If you are a spiritual person, pray about it. The answer will be made known to you.

Phlebotomy training

I am on a committee trying to establish updated guidelines for orientation and competency assessment in our lab. Occasionally, we are able to hire someone with training or experience, but most often it's off the street. What would be an appropriate length of time for training and any other guidelines you think would be useful?

The state of California mandates 80 hours of training followed by 50 supervised punctures and certification. Make that your goal. Anything less than 50 hours or so will manifest itself as unprofessional behavior, poor customer service skills, high specimen rejection rates, and poor technical expertise.

Reputable phlebotomy schools

I was wondering how I can find out if a school I am planning on attending is accredited.

One of the best indicators of a program's worth is its length. Some schools pretend to teach phlebotomy in a weekend, but a bona fide phlebotomy program, i.e., one that will be recognized as significant when it comes to looking for a job, should provide at least 50 hours of classroom time and the opportunity to do "clinicals." Clinicals are where students actually go to a hospital or other clinical setting and draw blood from real patients under the supervision of an experienced phlebotomist. Another good indicator of a reputable school is if they are accredited by the National Accrediting Agency for Clinical Laboratory Sciences (NAACLS). NAACLS accredits phlebotomy schools and other clinical laboratory courses. Visit www.naacls.org.

Student clinics

O ne of the requirements of our medical technology majors is a four-week course in phlebotomy that terminates with clinicals. One frequent concern of our students is that they don't feel prepared for the patients they would be drawing from, and that we should find a way to help them realize what to expect. How can we better prepare them for clinical patients?

F or students who have never been exposed to hospitalized patients, the shock of suddenly working on someone who is, for example, on a ventilator can be traumatic. You might consider recommending those who manage clinical rotations to start students off with a week of outpatients, then a week of low-acuity patients (e.g., OB patients), then work them into the more high-acuity/trauma patients. Keep in mind, the level of patient acuity is something mentors may not even know until they arrive with the student at the bedside.

Switching hands

I switch my hands after inserting the needle so that I can use my dominant hand to change tubes. My new supervisor insists I don't switch hands anymore. I am 50 years old and have ten years of experience, but now my hands are beginning to develop some arthritis. Following her suggestion would be more painful for me. Since I'm as proficient as anyone in the office, does my employer have the right to dictate what technique I use to hold the tube holder?

There is nothing in the standards or any text that prefers your employer's technique over yours, or vice versa. Which hand you use to change tubes is a matter of individual preference.

The one-handed technique your supervisor is suggesting (i.e., holding the tube holder with the same hand with which you insert the needle for the duration of the draw) is a good way to teach new phlebotomists who are less sure of themselves to draw blood. Those new to the procedure are more likely to dislodge the needle should they change hands in the middle of the draw. But for veteran phlebotomists like you who are comfortable with the switch, and can do so smoothly without displacing the needle, it sounds like an irrational request.

If you are just as successful as other phlebotomists who use the "same-hand" technique, there's no reason to make you change. Having said that, an employer can insist you follow facility policy, even if you disagree with that policy. To resist subjects you to charges of insubordination.

If it is the facility's policy to use the same-hand technique, then you ultimately have no choice. If you have addressed your concerns tactfully and diplomatically, and your employer still instructs you to use their method, there's not much you can do if you want to continue working there. If it boils down to either being right or being employed, it's your call. You sound like a very dedicated phlebotomist. Don't let this disagreement prevent you from continuing to provide quality patient care. Your patients need you.

Teaching hand-switching

I am a medical assistant instructor at a technical institute. One of our instructors is training our students to position the hand over the barrel when the needle is inserted into the vein, and then switch hands when the needle is inserted to work the tubes in and out of the tube holder. I am a little concerned because I have always heard that you are never to switch hands during a draw. Is it okay to train students to switch hands during a draw?

Asking a student to switch hands in the middle of a procedure that is already nerve-wracking enough invites needle dislocation and a failed attempt. It's just one too many steps to teach right from the beginning.

Many seasoned phlebotomists switch hands after the needle is in the vein to use their dominant hand to apply the tubes in and out of the holder. Teaching it to students, however, forces them to lose needle placement. They are usually so nervous and shaky that they don't dare let go of the needle, even to change hands. They need to focus on inserting the needle and keeping the hand steady and firmly supported on the patient's forearm throughout the draw.

If students later feel comfortable switching, that's up to them. The key is keeping the needle where they placed it. Making those new to the procedure switch hands is asking novices to adopt a technique only veteran stickers can execute without disrupting needle placement.

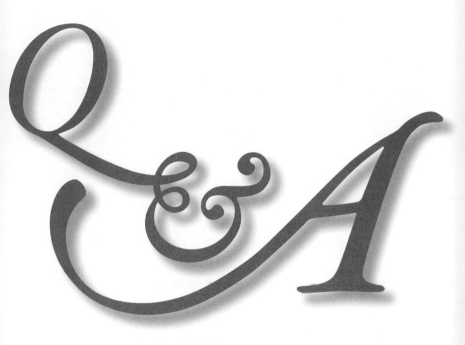

Decentralized phlebotomy

Our management has mentioned decentralizing phlebotomy as a money saving option. My current supervisor has worked at two facilities that tried decentralization, and they failed miserably. We want to focus on patient safety, patient identification, quality specimens, accurate results and competency. I need some references to help support centralized, not decentralized, phlebotomy.

There is lots of evidence in the literature about the downside of decentralization. Here are some references and article summaries:

1) Nelson, K. Recentralizing phlebotomy services in the clinical lab. *Adv Med Lab Prof* 2002;14(22):21–24.

This is an interesting hybrid model that worked successfully at the author's facility. The abstract of his article is available at www.Pubmed.com.

2) Savage R (ed). Q&A. *CAP Today* 1999;13(11):97–8.

This article (no longer archived on the CAP web site) is the editor's response to a reader's question in *CAP Today*'s Q&A column. The editor cites one hospital's nightmare with decentralization, reporting a 50% increase in their specimen rejection rate (210 to 300 per month) when nurses and clerks started performing phlebotomy. The article cites the following study as the source of that statistic: Gable J. Pyevac Z. Paradigm shift: phlebotomy belongs to nursing. *Clin Lab Mgmt Review*. 1995;9:286-297. The abstract is also at www.Pubmed.com.

3) Southwick K. Back to the drawing board: hospitals rethink their phlebotomy staffing practices. *CAP Today* 2001;15(2):12–18.

This article reports a tripling of the error rate due to unacceptable specimens when nurses draw blood as opposed to laboratory draws. You can find this article on the CAP web site: www.cap.org.

4) Jones B, Calam R, Howanitz P. Chemistry specimen acceptability. *Arch Pathol Lab Med* 1997;121:19–26.

This article showed that lab personnel submitted significantly fewer rejected specimens than other in-house non-lab personnel. The abstract is available on www.Pubmed.com.

5) Warner, J. Recentralizing phlebotomy back to the laboratory. *Clin Lab Mgmt Rev* 2005;19(4):E3.

The abstract of this article is also available on PubMed.

Did You Know...

the average phlebotomist commits 3.5 procedural errors per draw. (Source: Laboratory Medicine, March, 2002.)

Decentralized phlebotomy & failed venipuncture attempts

We have a decentralized phlebotomy service that constantly requires me to send up a lab-based phlebotomist for their "tough sticks." Having to pull our phlebotomist away from outpatient draws is a real drain on our resources and prevents nursing from taking full ownership of phlebotomy. What is considered a "reasonable" number of "tough stick" requests in a decentralized phlebotomy setting? I already believe that our rate is too high, but I don't quite know how to prove it.

A reasonable number of requests for your phlebotomist to leave the department to help with a tough stick on the floor is difficult to determine and unique to your facility. One study showed 95% of venipunctures performed by phlebotomists were successfully collected on first attempt; 2.8% required two attempts; 0.8% required three attempts and 1.1% required four or more sticks.[1] Unfortunately, this data is a bit dated, but it's a start.

Such a statistic is largely a function of many variables specific to the facility. Perhaps the only way to get a handle on it is to establish a list of acceptable reasons that draws get kicked back for the lab to perform. It's likely many of the draws you have to do are because the nurses don't have the time or don't have the confidence to be successful, but doing a survey of every request would be revealing. The problem will then be what to do with that information. On the other hand, what would be a valid reason to withhold your staff's expertise from the patient? It's a tough question that many facilities have to wrestle with.

Reference

1) Howantiz P, Schifman R. Inpatient phlebotomy practices: A College of American Pathologists Q-Probe study of 2,351,643 phlebotomy requests. *Arch Pathol Lab Med* 1994;118:601–605.

Decentralized phlebotomy stats

We currently have decentralized phlebotomy where clinical assistants draw the blood on all of our med/surg inpatients. Our customer satisfaction scores concerning inpatient phlebotomy draws are low. Our lab director is under the impression that the current trend is away from decentralized, towards centralized phlebotomy. Do you know of any published articles or data that discuss this issue?

Your director is correct. Most facilities that go to a decentralized phlebotomy service find their customer satisfaction surveys plummet. The problem is that there are insufficient resources allocated toward education of non-laboratory personnel to draw blood. Currently, the pendulum is swinging back towards centralizing phlebotomy to the laboratory again. However, some units are retaining the skill as a matter of necessity (i.e., ICU and ER).

Much has been written on the subject that should provide you with lots of information to help reclaim phlebotomy for your lab. Here's a summary for you:

1) Nelson, K. Recentralizing phlebotomy services in the clinical lab. *Adv. Med. Lab Prof* 2002;14(22):21–24.

2) Savage R (ed). Q&A. *CAP Today* 1999;13(11):97–8.

3) Southwick K. Back to the drawing board: hospitals rethink their phlebotomy staffing practices. *CAP Today* 2001;15(2):12–18.

4) Jones B, Calam R, Howanitz P. Chemistry specimen acceptability. *Arch Pathol Lab Med* 1997;121:19–26.

5) Warner, J. Recentralizing phlebotomy back to the laboratory. *Clin Lab Mgmt Rev* 2005;19(4):E3.

(cont...)

(Decentralized phlebotomy stats cont...)

The Nelson reference talks about an interesting hybrid model that worked successfully at the author's facility. The article is probably still archived at: http://laboratorian.advanceweb.com.

CAP Today no longer archives any issue prior to 2000, so that piece will be harder to find. The Jones reference is an article that showed lab personnel submitted significantly fewer rejected specimens than other in-house non-lab personnel. The abstract is available on www.Pubmed.com.

Jody Warner, author of the last reference above, gave a talk at a CLMA conference about how her facility was able to convince administration to reclaim phlebotomy as a laboratory procedure (recentralize). The abstract of her article is also available on PubMed.

Did You Know...

hospitals can save $20 per blood culture collected in reduced contamination rates if they train and assign a phlebotomy team as opposed to a multi-skilled workforce to draw blood cultures.

Disciplining phlebotomists

We have a veteran staff phlebotomist who has a chronic problem with recurring specimen collection errors. The errors are usually associated with incorrect specimen collections involving reference laboratory testing. At times, her error rate is up to 25%. She has a computer at her disposal for reference, but obviously does not utilize it.

———————————————————————⟨Ꭷ Ꮽ⟩————

There's a saying in human resource circles: "If they're worth keeping, they're worth correcting." I will assume you've corrected this person until you've run out of patience. She's probably a very nice lady, but if she's not taking you seriously, she's not taking her role in healthcare seriously, either.

It sounds to me that this person has no consequences for substandard performance. I would evaluate your management style with particular attention to how you discipline errors. Your patients, present and future, are depending on you to be their last line of defense against medication errors, specimen labeling errors, transfusion errors, misdiagnosis, and general medical mismanagement. It's time to be firm, and consider that someday, if she goes uncorrected, she could precipitate a medical mistake with disastrous consequences.

There should be a frank discussion about why she's been allowed to continue making mistakes with patient specimens, and apologies from you for being lenient. Explain why that tolerance is no longer going to be your way of managing the risk she's bringing to the facility. Make sure she understands why it is necessary to begin holding her to a higher standard, and provide new expectations of her performance.

Set benchmarks (e.g., 50% reduction in errors in 30 days, 75% in 60 days, etc.), and set the consequences for failing to meet the benchmarks (e.g., written warning followed by suspension followed by termination). But you have to make sure your benchmarks are not only for her, but that the rest of your staff meets them, too. You don't want to set higher standards for her than for everyone else.

(cont...)

(Disciplining phlebotomists cont...)

Put it all in writing so there's no misunderstanding. Then start a new day, one in which all past transgressions are forgotten and the only black marks on her record are those she puts there by not taking you seriously anymore.

Be prepared for her to challenge you. She'll want to see if you really are establishing higher standards or if you just needed to blow off steam. It is imperative that you implement your disciplinary measures just as you communicated. If you don't, you've lost her and others will soon drift to her level of performance.

A twenty-five percent error rate is enough to get most people fired. Few businesses that can survive with that kind of quality. It's not like she's making widgets. She's inviting medical mistakes that can have serious implications. Your concern is well placed.

Did You Know...
according to a Gallop poll, 19% of employees are "actively disengaged" at work.

Draws per hour

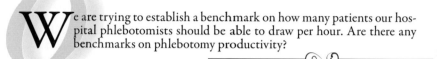

We are trying to establish a benchmark on how many patients our hospital phlebotomists should be able to draw per hour. Are there any benchmarks on phlebotomy productivity?

Because there are so many facility-dependent variables, you will be hard pressed to find phlebotomy productivity standards that can be universally and fairly applied. It would be best to establish your own workload productivity benchmark by conducting a small study that will take into effect all those variables that are unique to your facility, and that take into account the exact specifics of the procedure you want to include. Set up a study that times your staff in the performance of their regular duties according to the standards. Establish exactly when the procedure begins (e.g., time of the order, time the employee leaves the lab, the time they arrive at the patient's side.) Likewise, define the end of the procedure. Determine if you want to include fingersticks and heelsticks in the time study. Include a wide variety of personnel with a wide variety of experience at a wide range of times during the day. It wouldn't be fair to expect new phlebotomists to meet the productivity standard of seasoned personnel.

The March, 2003 issue of *Phlebotomy Today* has a nice article on specimen collection benchmarks, including productivity, frequency of bruising, average percent of venipunctures that are successful on the first attempt, etc. It is available as a download for a nominal fee at www.phlebotomy.com.

Interviewing new phlebotomists

I'm new in my position and I don't have very much experience in interviewing new phlebotomists. What can you tell me what to look for and ask about?

You need to evaluate new phlebotomists on at least three levels:

1.) How knowledgeable are they about phlebotomy? The more experience they have the easier they are to train. If they have experience, at least you know they are comfortable with the procedure and that they won't quit when they find out that phlebotomy isn't for them, as is the case sometimes with those new to the field. The downside to applicants having experience is that their experience may be in drawing blood incorrectly. If they weren't properly trained in the beginning, their experience may have only served to solidify poor technique. For them, breaking bad habits can be a challenge.

2.) How do they present themselves? Are they engaging in conversation? Are they pleasant and articulate? Are they professional in demeanor, manner and appearance? Don't forget, whoever you hire will project the only image of the lab many patients receive. One mistake many employers make is to hire on skill and experience alone, giving a low priority to character and integrity. You can teach the skill, but teaching values is a whole lot harder.

3.) How will they fit with the personalities and the nuances of your current staff? Will their personality clash or blend? Will they inspire or demoralize your staff? It can make the difference between a short-term and long-term employee. There are other factors to consider, but have a conversation with your human resources people to get more advice. They interview every day, and are very good at refining the process.

Maintaining competency

I'm a nurse in a public health unit, and I'm re-writing our medical directives for procedures done by RNs. The author of our current directives had decided that an individual who was trained, certified, and signed-off to perform phlebotomy needed to perform the procedure only once a year to maintain his/her competency. I took issue with this, and took on the task of trying to find recommendations by experts as to how frequently this skill should be implemented. Can you comment on this?

No one who draws one specimen a year can possibly maintain his/her skill. You are to be commended for upholding high standards for competency.

Although there are no established national standards on this topic, it's reasonable to suggest that to maintain competency a person should be drawing at least 3–5 patients a week. There's just too much to know that requires the reinforcement that only repetition at this rate can provide. Phlebotomy has been called the most underestimated procedure in healthcare. The assumption that one venipuncture per year is adequate to maintain competency reinforces that underestimation.

Minimum age for phlebotomists

I am the program director at a NAACLS accredited phlebotomy certificate program. We have had a couple of students apply to our program who graduated from high school early and are only 17 years old. I am trying to find documentation or regulations relating to an age limit for practicing phlebotomy. Can you assist with this matter?

To our knowledge, there really aren't any regulations limiting the age for phlebotomists. It's a highly unregulated profession. There may be limitations imposed by employers, but they're likely to only be general limitations and not specific to specimen collection personnel.

Outpatient drawing areas

D o you know whether a blood-drawing area can be shared with the rest of the lab processing area? The area another worker and I have for phlebotomy is very small. I also draw blood from infants. Is this okay?

A ccording to CLSI, venipuncture rooms should afford privacy during the blood collecting procedure. There may be a HIPAA requirement to assure patient confidentiality as well. Joint Commission has requirements on the amount of space that should be allocated to testing facilities, but space requirements for specimen processing or outpatient drawing areas may not be as well defined. You might look into their requirements for more guidance.

The final consideration is that patients must be protected from any biohazards. Does your facility have a policy that lab coats must be worn in the processing area? If so, drawing patients there might be problematic. Many labs do require lab coats in the processing area because exposure to blood and other infectious materials can be reasonably anticipated.

Phlebotomist salaries

I am attempting to increase the salary of our phlebotomists and would like some advice and/or help. Currently the starting salary for a new phlebotomist is $8.50. We cannot keep phlebotomists due to this low salary. Do you have any idea if this is within range of other hospitals our size (108 beds)?

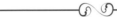

Salary surveys available at the time of publication show the average wage nationwide for phlebotomists to be $11.74. Compared to other hospitals your size, your wages are well below average ($11.06/hr). The median average for phlebotomists in rural hospitals is $10.00/hr. In your region, the median average for all phlebotomists was reported to be $10.33.

These are not starting salaries, but average salaries. Your starting salary ($8.50) is at the low end of the pay scale for what all phlebotomists earn.

Armed with this data, you might be able to negotiate a higher base rate with your administrators. If you could calculate the cost of your high turnover and convince them that a wage increase that results in a decreased turnover would save the hospital money that would be even more compelling. Figure out how much you are spending in advertising for, interviewing, and training new employees per year. It's all about lost productivity.

But consider that it may not all be about money to your phlebotomists. Do they feel appreciated? If not, address the issues. Designate a day during Lab Week as Phlebotomist Appreciation Day. Launch a campaign informing all hospital employees how important the phlebotomist is to accurate results and, hence, patient care.

It's hard to change perceptions in small healthcare environments because you probably have a large percentage of hospital employees who have been there a long time and whose impressions of phlebotomists are deeply rooted. But that's no reason to accept them as permanent.

Do your phlebotomists act professionally? If not, it will be hard to get the rest of the hospital to respect them and, hence, hard to get them to feel respected. So maybe it's time to nurture a culture of professionalism by setting a Code of Conduct that includes phone etiquette, a dress code, what's considered unacceptable behavior, customer service tips, etc.

Do you encourage certification? If the hospital would pay the application fee, would your staff become certified? Nothing makes one feel professional like becoming certified in the field. Once the staff is certified, they are much more likely to gain the respect of other healthcare professions in the field.

Did You Know...

the cost to employers of dissatisfied
employees is $292-355 billion per year.

Phlebotomy awards

A re there any nationally recognized service awards for phlebotomy teams?

P hlebotomy is a largely underappreciated and unrecognized profession. That needs to change. If phlebotomists had their own membership organization, that would really help bring them recognition. They'd be able to develop the kinds of programs you're discussing. You might contact the major laboratory membership organizations and urge them to establish some kind of phlebotomy team recognition award.

Proper way to hold a tube holder

I am the phlebotomy manager at a healthcare facility in New York. I'm wondering if NAACLS states in their standards what the correct hold is for the tube-holder assembly. We seem to have some conflicting opinions in our area.

B efore addressing your question, I need to clear up some confusion. NAACLS does not publish the standards; they accredit clinical laboratory programs. The standards are published by the Clinical and Laboratory Standards Institute (CLSI). The confusion is understandable because CLSI used to be NCCLS.

CLSI doesn't get that specific about how a tube holder should be held. Much of it is personal preference. Most seasoned phlebotomists hold the tube holder like a pool cue, i.e., at the tips of the fingers. Two or three fingers are under the tube holder and the thumb is on top. This allows plenty of room to maneuver the tubes in and out, plus it allows you to rest the backs of your fingers on the patient's forearm for support.

Recollects & bruising benchmarks

I suspect some of our staff aren't very skilled at drawing based on recollects and the extent of bruising. Is there anything out there that suggests the average number of bruises and recollects per phlebotomist?

There aren't any published stats on bruises and recollects per phlebotomist, but there are statistics per patient. The March, 2004 issue of *Phlebotomy Today* (available as a download at www.phlebotomy.com), contains a comprehensive review of the literature. In summary, it cites a CAP Q-Probe published in 1991 that examined patient satisfaction and complications among 30,000 patients.[1] The average size of a bruise from a venipuncture was found to be 15.1 mm and the frequency of bruising was determined to be 16.1 percent of all venipunctures performed.

In terms of recollects, the number of attempts by phlebotomists per patient averaged 1.03. A second study addressed the level of recollects at 70 hospitals.[2] Ninety-five percent were collected on first attempt; 2.8% required two attempts; 0.8% required three attempts and 1.1% required four or more sticks.

These studies considered laboratory draws, not draws in a decentralized environment, and are a bit dated. A study in 2002 showed a 99.6 percent successful-draw rate for laboratory-managed collectors versus 97.9 percent when specimens were drawn by non-laboratory personnel.[3] This study is more current, but measured recollects for a wide variety of reasons besides failure to access the vein.

If you're looking for information on recollects due to specimen rejection, some current data exists here, too. One study reported non-laboratory personnel had a significantly higher specimen rejection rate than laboratory personnel.[4] Some facilities have reported a doubling and tripling of rejected specimens when nursing personnel were given blood collection responsibilities.[5] Other articles report an increase in monthly rejected specimens from 210 to 300 when the nursing staff took over phlebotomy duties.[6]

References

1) Howantiz P, Cembrowski G, Bachner P. Laboratory phlebotomy. *Arch Pathol Lab Med* 1991;115:867–872.

2) Howantiz P, Schifman R. Inpatient phlebotomy practices: A College of American Pathologists Q-Probe study of 2,351,643 phlebotomy requests. *Arch Pathol Lab Med* 1994;118:601–605.

3) Dale J, Novis D. Outpatient phlebotomy success and reasons for specimen rejection. *Arch Pathol Lab Med* 2002;126:416–9.

4) Jones B, Calam R, Howantiz P. Chemistry specimen acceptability; a CAP Q-Probes study of 703 laboratories. *Arch Pathol Lab Med* 1997;121:19–26.

5) Southwick, K. Back to the drawing board: Hospitals rethink their phlebotomy staffing practices. *CAP Today* **2001;15(2):12–18**.

6) Savage R (Editor) Q&A. *CAP Today* 1999;13(11):97–8.

Redraw rates

W hen our hospital-wide phlebotomy program was instituted several years ago, we set a QA redraw rate threshold of 1.5% for the phlebotomies performed by nurses and nurse technicians. It's currently running at 2.0% versus 0.15% for lab assistant/phlebotomist draws. Do you have any data or information on benchmarks for redraws?

⎯⎯⎯⎯⎯⎯⎯⎯⎯⎯⎯ Ꭷ Ꭷ ⎯⎯

W hen you look into the stats for redraw rates, there are two sets of data you must consider separately: redraws due to failed attempts, and redraws due to rejected specimens. In both cases, studies favor laboratory-based specimen collection personnel.

A CAP Q-Probe conducted in 1992 addressed the level of recollects at 683 hospitals and found that 95% of venipunctures performed by laboratory personnel were successful on the first attempt; 2.8% required two attempts; 0.8% required three attempts and 1.1% required four or more sticks.[1] (Although non-laboratory personnel were not included in either study, this statistic will provide you with a benchmark for laboratory draws. The study is a bit dated, but I still think there's something that can be learned from it.) A second study showed a 99.6% successful-draw rate for laboratory-managed collectors versus 97.9% when specimens were drawn by non-laboratory personnel.[2]

Non-laboratory personnel also show a significant increase in specimen rejection rates.[3] Some facilities experience a doubling, even a tripling, of rejected specimens when drawn by nursing personnel.[4] Other researchers have reported an increase in rejected specimens per month from 210 to 300 when nurses and clerks began performing phlebotomy.[5]

References

1) Howantiz P, Schifman R. Inpatient phlebotomy practices: A College of American Pathologists Q-Probe study of 2,351,643 phlebotomy requests. *Arch Pathol Lab Med* 1994;118:601–605.3

2) Dale J, Novis D. Outpatient phlebotomy success and reasons for specimen rejection. *Arch Pathol Lab Med* 2002;126:416–9.4

3) Jones B, Calam R, Howantiz P. Chemistry specimen acceptability; a CAP Q-Probes study of 703 laboratories. *Arch Pathol Lab Med* 1997;121:19–26.

4) Southwick, K. Back to the drawing board: Hospitals rethink their phlebotomy staffing practices. *CAP Today* **2001;15(2):12–18**.

5) Savage R (Editor) Q&A. *CAP Today* 1999;13(11):97–8.

Did You Know...
46% to 56% of all specimen errors occur during the collection or processing phase.

I drew an extra tube of blood for a potential type and crossmatch to keep a patient from having to be stuck a fourth time on the same day. The type & cross was never ordered. When administration heard that I drew the tube without written request, I was written up and given a five-day suspension. I think that's excessive. What do you think?

For patients in emergency settings, phlebotomists usually are encouraged to draw extra tubes on patients with existing orders, not punished. It's called being proactive. Such forward thinking often saves critical time when patient results warrant immediate physician intervention. Drawing blood for tests not ordered when no orders exist at all, however, is performing an unnecessary venipuncture that puts patients at an unnecessary risk. Disciplinary measures would then be justifiably taken. Any recourse you might have depends on if you violated a written policy against the practice.

You didn't mention if you were drawing from an emergency room patient or not, but regardless, your punishment seems harsh. Suspension for a first time offense like this, one that has no potential for adverse patient outcomes, does seem excessive. There must be more to the story than this, given the severity of the action.

You might consider contacting the Human Resource department to see if your suspension reflects facility policy. Other than that, you might contact the state's labor relations board to inquire what, if any, recourse an unjustifiably suspended employee might have.

Workload productivity

I follow the hand-washing procedure that states we are to wash our hands and change our gloves between each patient. Because my coworkers don't wash their hands between patients, they are able to draw more patients than I am.

I draw seven to eight patients per hour. I'm told that I need to draw the national average of 10 to 12 or else! Yet nobody can produce proof of this "national average." Can you tell me if such an average exists?

A study done in 1991 showed that the median time required for phlebotomy in 630 institutions was six minutes.[1] Twenty-five percent of the patients required less than five minutes while 10% required more than 21 minutes. Keep in mind that the study is based on practices in place prior to the issuance of the Bloodborne Pathogens Standard, which required handwashing after glove removal. Handwashing today is also required by the CLSI standards, and is probably mandated in your facility's own policy manual.[2]

It would be reasonable to expect that the average time for a phlebotomy is closer to seven minutes; that's if everything goes smoothly and all the standards are met. It sounds like you work for a "quantity-not-quality" facility. It's not likely your pleas for compliance are going to fall on compassionate hearts.

References

1) Howanitz P, Cembrowski G, Bachner P. Laboratory Phlebotomy: College of American Pathologists Q-Probe study of patient satisfaction and complications in 23,783 patients. *Arch Pathol Lab Med* 1991:115;867–72.

2) CLSI. *Procedures for the Collection of Diagnostic Blood Specimens by Venipuncture; Approved Standard—Sixth Edition.* CLSI document H3-A6. Wayne, PA: Clinical and Laboratory Standards Institute; 2007.

Certification, Canada

Q I have noticed that in the U.S. a phlebotomist can be certified. Can one be certified in Canada as well? Also, is there any online continuing education on any Canadian web sites?

A It's difficult to tell a web site's country of origin, but it shouldn't matter as long as the online education is accurate.

As for certification, any of the reputable certification organizations would certify you regardless of where you live, but the question is whether or not your employer would recognize it. Perhaps you are not so much concerned that your employer would recognize it as you are to better yourself. That's commendable. I don't think any certification agency would refuse to certify you just because you are not in the states. Visit www.phlebotomy.com for a list of recommended certification agencies, and pose that question to any or all of them.

Certification,
grandfathering in by experience

When I suggested to my boss that one day every phlebotomist would need to be certified, he laughed and said that would never happen. He said that if it did, everyone would just be grandfathered in. Is that true?

One of the sadder truths about phlebotomy is that only three states have any regulations whatsoever mandating certification or minimum training (California, Louisiana, and Nevada). Other states are considering it, but legislation takes a long time and passionate commitments from people like you. If legislation ever becomes enacted in your state, there is no guarantee there will be a grandfathering clause, or to what extent current phlebotomists would be grandfathered. When California enacted their legislation for example, all phlebotomists had to take a 20-hour program and a certification exam. Those who didn't have experience had to take an 80-hour program and pass an exam. I commend you on finding value in certification and hope your passion and pride in the profession spreads throughout your staff.

Certification: is it required to draw blood?

Q I am a Certified Respiratory Therapist. Recently I began working in a doctor's office where the physician wants me to draw blood. Do I have to be licensed or certified other than as an RT?

A You only need to become certified if you live in California, Nevada, and to a lesser extent, Louisiana. Anywhere else, you can learn on the job without formal training. Hard to believe, but it's true. Because phlebotomy is a highly detailed procedure and not at all as easy as it looks, it would behoove you to pursue training outside your facility. Patients can be permanently injured from poorly performed venipunctures. Having said that, your office staff might be very adept at performing venipunctures and might be capable of training you properly with attention paid to things like the order of draw, minimum fill volumes, high-risk veins of the antecubital area, proper angle of insertion, limits to needle manipulation, etc.

I would consider undergoing a formal training program, maybe at your local community college or at an approved phlebotomy school. You can find links to several school directories at www.phlebotomy.com. Even though certification may not be required, it's a good idea. A lot can go wrong and most people underestimate the procedure.

Legislation

I'm looking for a list of all the states that require licensure/certification and what, if any, other requirements are necessary in those states. We plan on hiring phlebotomists throughout the US and this information would be very helpful.

*C*alifornia has the most comprehensive and sweeping legislation. They require 80 hours of training, 50 successful venipunctures and successful completion by a state-approved certification agency. For more information, visit: https://secure.cps.ca.gov/cltreg.

Nevada requires those who draw blood in licensed laboratories be certified as laboratory assistants. Nevada labs can call them "phlebotomists" if they want, but as far as the state's concerned, they must be certified laboratory assistants to draw blood. Specimen collection personnel in physicians' offices are exempt if the physician provides documentation of experience. For more information on Nevada's legislation, see the revised statute NRS 652.127 at: www.leg.state.nv.us.

Louisiana has some legislation on the books, but it exempts nearly all clinical lab employees who are under the direct supervision of a laboratory tech, nurse or physician. The only other state considering legislation at the time of publication is Massachusetts.

The value of certified phlebotomists

If a phlebotomist has gained certification, how much should that add to his/her worth to an organization?

The value of certification to an organization depends upon who gets to ascribe it. How do you put a number on the higher morale a certified work force often demonstrates over a non-certified staff? What is the value of the patient's impression when a facility is staffed with certified phlebotomists versus non-certified? The value of certification is really immeasurable, and a function of the organization's perception of the value of certification. Some organizations consider it to have little value, to others it's significant. There are too many intangibles to give it a dollar amount.

A CEO may find certification to be of no value only because it cannot be translated into increased revenue, yet the manager of the specimen collection staff may find it to be of immeasurable value because she doesn't have the recollection issues and customer service headaches that she did with a non-certified staff.

In our opinion, from a monetary standpoint, certified phlebotomists should earn at least 20% more in their hourly rate than non-certified phlebotomists. From the standpoint of what certification can mean to a person's sense of pride and professionalism, their longevity in the workplace, a sense of ownership of the procedure, and self-worth is worth more than anyone can possibly afford to pay.

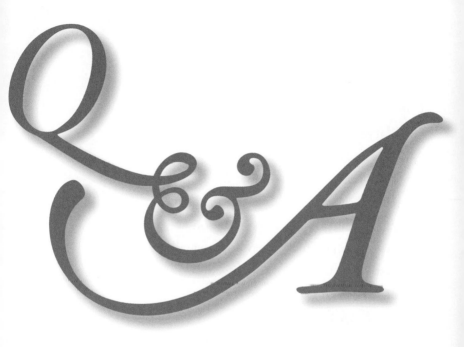

3. Skin Punctures, Heelsticks, & Pain Management

Skin Punctures/Heelsticks

Age limit on venipunctures

Alcohol and fingersticks

Analyte differences between capillary and venous blood

Capillary punctures and mastectomies

Capillary sticks on all fingers

Clotting and capillary collections

Crying babies

Fingerstick site and first-drop elimination

Fingersticks, depth of skin penetration

Fingersticks on infants old enough to walk

Fingersticks to the side of the finger

Infant heelsticks: lateral versus plantar

Minimum age for fingersticks

Nurses and fingersticks

Orientation of the heelstick device

Performing infant fingersticks

Skin punctures to the big toe

Pain Management

Administering oral sucrose to outpatients

EMLA and other topical anesthetics

Heel warmers vs. warm towels or warm water gloves

Heelstick, depth of puncture

Pain management

Prewarming

Skin punctures through bruised heels

Age limit on venipunctures

What is your recommendation on obtaining blood from children under two years old? Should fingersticks be done? We currently do arm sticks when possible. We do heelsticks on infants.

The latest CLSI skin puncture and venipuncture standards don't state whether skin punctures or venipunctures are recommended on children under two years of age. However, the skin puncture standard states when performing a skin puncture on infants up to 12 months of age, the heel is the only recommended site. On infants older than 12 months, fingersticks are the recommended site because heels at that age are too thick and less likely to yield adequate volumes.

Venipunctures are acceptable for any age when more blood is required than can be obtained from a skin puncture. However, they carry a risk. If the venipuncture is performed in children without verbal skills, the collector has no way of knowing when he/she may have come in contact with a nerve; all screams sound alike. The risk is especially acute when drawing from the basilic vein on the inside (medial) aspect of the antecubital area. Having said that, an article citing three separate studies reported that venipunctures on infants were less painful than heelsticks.[1]

Reference

1) Franck AL, Gilbert R. Reducing pain during blood sampling in infants. *Clin Evid* 2002. Jun;(7):352–66.

Alcohol and fingersticks

Please let me know the latest on using alcohol wipes for fingersticks, especially for glucose meters. Is alcohol an interfering substance?

Alcohol is fine for all fingersticks as long as it is allowed to dry first. I know of no study that has found it to interfere with any routinely performed fingerstick test. If wet, it can hemolyze red cells, but if it is allowed to dry, there should be no interference.

Analyte differences between capillary and venous blood

Do you have any studies that show the differences in results between samples collected by venipuncture and those collected by fingerstick? We are primarily concerned with CBCs. My experience is that a venipuncture is the preferred method.

The thinking that blood obtained by venipuncture renders a more accurate representation of the patient's circulating blood than that obtained by skin puncture is disputable. This conception may be based on the presumption that all venipunctures are performed correctly and cleanly and all capillary punctures are contaminated by hemolysis and tissue fluids. Although the latter concern may be justified, when properly performed, skin punctures can render a sample just as representative of the circulation as that obtained by venipuncture. (Note: skin punctures or incisions performed on edematous sites or from dehydrated patients may not yield representative results regardless of technique.)

Nevertheless, there are some known differences between the composition of venous and capillary blood. Capillary specimens show lower concentrations of sodium, chloride, potassium, total protein, bilirubin, and calcium and higher concentrations of glucose.[1,2] Researchers advise against considering venous glucose and capillary glucose equivalent when it comes to managing diabetes.[3] Capillary samples tend to run about eight percent higher in glucose than venipuncture samples after a meal or ingesting a loading dose of glucose. But for random or fasting glucose determinations, venous plasma glucose is higher than capillary glucose. Glucose in plasma has been found to be 14–16 percent higher than in whole blood.

References

1) CLSI. *Procedures and Devices for the Collection of Diagnostic Capillary Blood Specimens; Approved Standard—Sixth Edition.* CLSI document H4-A6. Wayne, PA: Clinical and Laboratory Standards Institute; 2008.

2) Baer D (ed).Tips from the Clinical Experts. *MLO* 2008;40(3):50–51.

3) Clinical Abstracts. Use of vein vs capillary blood as samples. *CAP Today* 2005;19(2):109.

Did You Know...
punctures on the fingers should be done
across the fingerprint, not parallel to them.

Capillary punctures and mastectomies

I read an article in *Phlebotomy Today* that a capillary puncture should never be performed on the same side as a mastectomy. I had never heard this before. Could you please let me know the rationale behind this so I may instruct our employees in the proper technique? We are currently doing finger-sticks on both hands regardless of history of mastectomy.

According to CLSI—the organization that sets the standards—finger-sticks are off limits on the same side as a mastectomy without physician's permission. The standard cites the American Cancer Society's website.[1] The rationale is that any trauma to the affected side can result in infection and lead to lymphedema. That's why we prefer to let the physician make the call and assume the liability.

Reference

1) CLSI. *Procedures and Devices for the Collection of Diagnostic Capillary Blood Specimens; Approved Standard—Sixth Edition.* CLSI document H4-A6. Wayne, PA: Clinical and Laboratory Standards Institute; 2008.

2) Brennan MJ, Weitz J. Lymphedema 30 years after radical mastectomy. *Am J Phys Med Rehabil* 1992 Feb;71(1):12–4.

3) HIV Counseling, Testing & Referral Program Quarterly Newsletter. Oct./Nov. 2006. Missouri Department of Health and Senior Services. http://www.dhss.mo.gov/HIV_AIDS/4thQ2006.pdf. Accessed 6/20/08.

4) OncoLink. Abramson Cancer Center at the University of Pennsylvania. http://www.oncolink.org/experts/article.cfm?c=3&s=13&ss=22&id=2046. Accessed 6/20/08.

5) Ask an Expert. The Johns Hopkins Breast Cancer Center website. http://www.hopkinsbreastcenter.org/services/ask_expert/index.asp?cat=23&pagenum=3. Accessed 6/20/08.

Capillary sticks on all fingers

I have recently been working with our nursing staff to make sure they are performing capillary punctures for bedside glucose testing according to CLSI standards. Because many of our patients are stuck several times a day over a period of several days (especially our tight glycemic-control patients), the nurses are concerned that using only the middle and ring fingers will not provide a sufficient number of sites for these patients. I have given them a copy of the standard, which gives reasons why the thumb, forefinger, and little finger should not be used, but they're still saying it's just not practical in the real world. What should I tell them?

Not practical? Giving the patient gangrene because the sharp penetrated the bone of the little finger is not practical. Having the patient bleed profusely because they punctured the artery in the thumb is not practical. Testifying to a jury on why they thought they could defy the standards is not practical.

Tell them that standards are standards for a reason and if they want to operate outside of the standard of care they should do so for another employer. Of course, you'll need to be more diplomatic than that, but I have seen dozens upon dozens of cases in which patients were permanently injured because someone wanted to defy the procedure. So there's little room for patience when it comes to arguing against the standard of care. If they don't want to do it right and if they don't want to follow facility policy, they shouldn't do it at all.

Clotting and capillary collections

Is there anything special about the collection of skin-puncture specimens from PICU and NICU? Some of our larger facilities have clotting issues with these types of collections. Any thoughts?

Babies' hematocrits are usually high, but that shouldn't make specimens clot faster. Mixing during collection is critical. If collectors wait until the specimen is filled, then mix, the EDTA tube will likely be clotted. Mixing the tube periodically during collection rather than waiting until after the tube is filled. This can be done by tapping the device gently on a hard surface. If the collection tube is a closed system (e.g., drawn through a straw protruding through a sealed closure), then you might successfully mix the anticoagulant with the blood by gently flicking the bottom of the tube. But don't try this on an open system, since splatter is likely. Cap and invert all specimens thoroughly after collection.

A lengthy draw delays mixing by inversion, so I would also suggest prewarming the heel before the draw. It increases blood flow through the capillary beds seven fold. Without prewarming, collection can take a lot longer and require excessive squeezing.

Prewarming takes 3–5 minutes. About the same amount of time as it takes to squeeze enough hemolyzed blood out of an infant's heel that has not been prewarmed. If your staff implements these two techniques, then they shouldn't have a problem.

Crying babies

I have a phlebotomist who keeps telling people that letting a child cry helps them bleed better. I do not find any source to back this up and honestly I do not believe there is any truth behind it. Can you clear this up for me?

Crying makes a baby bleed better? We're not sure about that one. You won't find anything in any reputable publication or standard to support this quirky idea. What we do know is that crying elevates the white count. Perhaps it would be a good idea to scrutinize the individual's technique for other such contrived ideas about drawing blood.

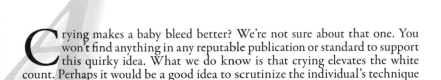

Fingerstick site and first-drop elimination

There's an issue brewing between our diabetes educator and our point-of-care coordinator concerning wiping away the first drop of blood after a fingerstick before blood is tested. Neither the educator nor the manufacturer of the glucose meter instructs this step. What do the standards say? Also, the glucose meter manufacturer's info recommends the side of the finger for the puncture, which is what the educator is teaching as well. I teach phlebotomy students according to CLSI recommendations, which is to use the fleshy pad of the finger. Who's right?

As for the site of the fingerstick, you are correct that the meter's manufacturer is making a recommendation that is in direct conflict with the CLSI standards. I would contact them and ask them why the discrepancy. By advocating such contrary practices, it makes your job infinitely more difficult, and opens your facility up to liability should any puncture to the (thinner) side of the finger result in bone penetration and the complications that can arise, not the least of which is gangrene and amputation. Attorneys have a much easier case to prosecute when procedures that led to patient injury are found to be in direct violation of the standards. I'd bring your risk manager in on this.

As far as first-drop elimination, one must consider that the first drop contains tissue fluid from the trauma of the puncture, which can dilute the results, making them falsely lower. But it's important to always follow the instrument manufacturer's instructions on the use of the equipment. Perhaps the device is calibrated and the reference range is established on the first drop. The manufacturer should be allowed to defend their recommendation on both accounts.

Fingersticks, depth of skin penetration

I'm looking for some new lancets, and wonder what the CLSI guidelines are for fingerstick puncture depth. I know the standard for heelsticks is to puncture no deeper than 2.0 mm, but none of my phlebotomists are happy with the return of blood from a fingerstick puncture at that depth. Are there guidelines about performing deeper punctures based on the patient's age?

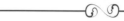

As you probably know, fingersticks are not recommended unless the infant is at least a year old, so let's assume your question is about older patients. Keep in mind the 2.0 mm penetration limit recommended by CLSI is only for the heels of infants. Fingers of older children and adults are more tolerant. Still, charts recommending various puncture depths as a function of age don't exist. Tissue depth at the fingertips is so widely diverse that it wouldn't be prudent. CLSI references the following articles in its passage on skin puncture depth:

1) Reiner CB, Meites S, Hayes JR. Optimal sites and depths for specimens by skin puncture of infants and children as assessed from anatomical measurements. *Clin Chem* 1990;36:547–549.

2) Blumenfeld TA, Turi GK, Blanc WA. Recommended sites and depth of newborn heel skin punctures based on anatomic measurements and histopathology. *Lancet* 1979;1:213.

I would suggest your phlebotomists increase the volume of blood from the puncture site by prewarming the heel or finger for 3–5 minutes prior to the puncture. Prewarming increases the flow of blood through the capillary beds by seven fold. That's pretty significant. Not only does prewarming give you more volume, but the specimen is cleaner and less likely to be contaminated by tissue fluid from excessive milking of the site.

Fingersticks on infants old enough to walk

We have read some articles that say once a child is walking, the heel should no longer be used regardless of the infant's age. Yet other articles strictly prohibit fingersticks unless the child is twelve months or older. Some walking infants get pretty strong by the time they are 12 months old and can kick like crazy. Is the 12-month rule really that hard and fast?

You are wise to be skeptical about any article that says heelsticks shouldn't be performed on infants who are walking. It goes against the CLSI standard, which states that fingersticks should not be performed on infants less than 12 months of age. The concern is with bone penetration. Just because the infant walks, doesn't mean the finger is thick enough for a skin puncture. If you use a prewarming technique on the heels of ambulatory infants less than a year old, you shouldn't have difficulty getting the sample.

Fingersticks to the side of the finger

One of our NAs (nursing assistants) stated that she was taught to perform the stick on the side of the finger, not the pad. Now she's teaching this to other NAs. When I brought this up to the clinical educator, she stated they were trained to do that as a way of avoiding tender finger pads. CLSI specifically states that the side of the finger is not acceptable due to lack of tissue between skin and bone. She refuses to change unless the American Diabetes Association (ADA) says the side is not acceptable. This puts me in a tight spot. The ADA web site says nothing about the collection procedures. What do I do?

Since when do employees get to negotiate their compliance with facility policy? Since the NA wants to go against facility policy, the burden of proof should be on her, not you. Ask for documentation that backs up her stance. She won't find it.

It's likely the ADA doesn't address the technical aspects of specimen collection because they know there is already an agency with authority in the field, namely CLSI. Tell the NA that specimen collection techniques are not addressed by the ADA, and that your facility policy is based on CLSI standards. Mention that failure to comply with facility policy puts the facility at risk of liability and patients at risk of injury. It also constitutes insubordination. Mention that you simply can't allow individuals to reinvent well-established procedures, especially when they are in contradiction to nationally recognized standards. If she doesn't want to comply, she simply should not be allowed to teach or perform procedures contrary to the facility's established procedure.

Hard telling what other specimen collection techniques she doesn't agree with and is misleading other NAs about. You don't want to start a war here, but you don't want to put patients at risk of injury, or the facility at risk of litigation. Bring your risk manager into the conversation. Perhaps if the educator won't listen to you, the risk manager will have more influence.

Infant heelsticks: lateral versus plantar

A couple of the nurses in a local hospital are directing our phlebotomists to perform punctures on the lateral surface of the heel rather than the plantar surface. We are familiar with the CLSI guidelines and instruct students in accordance with those guidelines, emphasizing punctures to the plantar surface of the heel. Would you be kind enough to comment on the nurses' practice and any adverse affects that may occur?

Typically, the plantar surface of the heel refers to the bottom of the heel, i.e., the surface of the heel that one might stand on. Taber's Medical Dictionary refers to the plantar surface as the "sole of the foot." The CLSI skin puncture standard recommends the lateral or medial plantar surface of the heel. The lateral or medial plantar surface, therefore, would be the sides of the heel, but not the back. If you have this CLSI document (H4-A6), you can see an illustration of the locations that are acceptable. Most texts also have an illustration. So when the nurses say the lateral surface of the heel, they are correct. But you wouldn't want to puncture way up the side, of course.

Minimum age for fingersticks

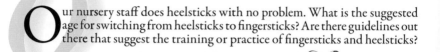

Our nursery staff does heelsticks with no problem. What is the suggested age for switching from heelsticks to fingersticks? Are there guidelines out there that suggest the training or practice of fingersticks and heelsticks?

The standards for the practice of fingersticks and heelsticks are established by the Clinical and Laboratory Standards Institute (CLSI). It states that fingersticks should not be done on infants less than 1 year of age. Their fingers are so tiny that bone penetration could occur and lead to gangrene, septicemia, and complications that could include amputation, even death.

As for training, there are no minimum requirements as to the extent of instruction other than those in effect in the states of California and Nevada at the time of publication. This is unfortunate because many patients suffer from medical mismanagement from poorly performed phlebotomy procedures due to the lack of regulation. It's important that healthcare professionals don't underestimate the importance of proper and comprehensive training.

Nurses and fingersticks

We are a community-based hospital with decentralized phlebotomy. Our LPNs do the draws on the units, then the blood is delivered to the laboratory for analysis. When the draw is difficult, they call the lab to send up a phlebotomist. We want to investigate the possibility of having the LPNs do fingersticks to obtain the specimen if the venipuncture has failed instead of waiting for the lab phlebotomist. Do you have any information about nurses doing fingersticks? Is it a common practice for the same person who missed a vein to do a fingerstick?

There are no restrictions or regulations (outside of California, Nevada, and Louisiana) on who can perform a venipuncture or capillary puncture. It is up to the facility to train their staff properly so that the procedure is done correctly and does not compromise the integrity of the specimen or the quality of patient care. This is no small task since the specimen is so vulnerable to change based on collection and processing practices.

Skin punctures can be a valid alternative to venipunctures if the tests can be performed on minimal volumes. Some analytes vary between capillary and venous blood, so your laboratory should take that into consideration when reporting results. Most who perform venipunctures are also skilled and trained in capillary punctures. But again, it's up to the employer to properly train the collector to perform the procedure so that the specimen reflects the patient's physiology. If poorly performed, or if performed without a knowledge of the standards for blood specimen collection, the specimen can be substantially altered so that the test result leads the physician to mismanage the patient.

Orientation of the heelstick device

For the past week, our lab has been discussing the proper method to use when performing infant heelsticks. There's one lingering question that we can't seem to find an answer to. When many of us were trained, we were trained to keep the incision perpendicular rather than parallel to the length of the foot. Now that we are in the process of re-writing policies and competency testing, we can't find a thing in writing supporting one method over another. Does it really matter?

There is nothing in the literature (i.e., textbooks, standards, or any other authoritative treatise) that favors one orientation over another. Manufacturers may recommend one way, but no rationale is given. Most specimen collection personnel perform a puncture parallel with the foot, but it may be only a matter of habit. It's more important that the punctures are on the proper locations of the heel than any particular orientation within those acceptable areas. You're free to write your policy any way you choose.

Performing infant fingersticks

Currently, our pediatric policy for the hospital states that any child weighing less than 22 lbs. will have a heel stick. The phlebotomists say that these babies are big and healthy and they are finding it hard to wrap their hand around their heel. They also complain that their kick is really strong and they are ending up with clotted specimens. Are there any guidelines concerning fingersticks on babies between 18–22 lbs.? What lancet depth would be appropriate to use if a fingerstick was performed?

According to the CLSI guideline, fingersticks are not allowed on infants less than one year old. For older infants, no depth is given for fingersticks. Companies that manufacture fingerstick devices usually have devices with a variety of depths. Some penetrate to a depth of 0.85 mm.

If your phlebotomists take the time to prewarm the heels of infants, they would likely get a better blood flow. It's not advisable to allow them to go against the standards and perform fingersticks just because the heel is too big. If the blade penetrates to the bone of the finger, complications including gangrene can make it a regrettable deviation.

Skin punctures to the big toe

I have clinics that are performing capillary sticks for hemoglobin testing in the doctors' offices. They currently use the big toe on six-month olds. Nowhere in the literature am I able to reference the great toe as an acceptable site. Please advise what the appropriate practice is in this case.

In prior versions of the CLSI skin puncture standard, the great toe was included as a recommended site. However, in 2004, it was removed from the list because heels provide such a sufficient number of options that the great toe needn't be "recommended."

With that in mind, there is nothing wrong with performing a skin puncture on the great toe, nor are there risks that would make it unacceptable. The reason you aren't finding it in the literature anymore is because reputable texts reflect CLSI's standards.

Administering oral sucrose to outpatients

What is the latest on using sucrose for pain management for infant collection? Since sucrose is a food substance, can it be administered to infants in an outpatient draw area? OSHA doesn't allow food to be consumed in the laboratory, so is this even legal?

Many studies have shown oral sweeteners to reduce pain responses during infant heel puncture and venipuncture, particularly the duration of crying. The larger issue is about who is allowed to administer oral sweeteners to infants.

For inpatients, it's a nursing decision and responsibility. For outpatient infants, it should be the mother's. Most facilities won't allow phlebotomists to administer such fluids, as it is not in their scope of practice nor part of the procedure. It's common for labs to administer glucose beverages in the outpatient area to patients undergoing a glucose tolerance test, so there's a precedent already set for infants to consume oral sweeteners as a method of pain prevention. Nevertheless, facilities need to consider all the facets of this practice and come up with their own policies.

The issue of consuming it in clinical areas is not an OSHA issue, however. OSHA guidelines only apply to employers and employees, not patients.

EMLA and other topical anesthetics

We are considering a policy on using topical anesthetics (like EMLA®) for venipuncture pain. The mother of one of our pediatric patients says it helps her son handle the digging. Do you know what other facilities have in the way of procedures for such ointments? Does it require a doctor's order?

The mother's comment that EMLA makes it easier for her son to "handle the digging" is a chilling statement. EMLA might prevent the initial sting, but it won't prevent a permanent nerve injury, which can and has happened when those who draw specimens think digging is acceptable.

EMLA® and other topical anesthetics may have their place, but there's no substitute for compassion and good technique when it comes to drawing pediatrics. Unfortunately, some who put topical anesthetics in their arsenal do so too quickly. Just make sure such approaches are your last resort, not your first.

One of a child's greatest fears is the fear of the unknown. To defuse this fear, one only needs to invest a little prep time in some compassionate "kidspeak." Most apprehensive children (but not all) can be calmed by lowering oneself down to the child's eye level and explaining the procedure. Walking through the steps and simulating what the tourniquet will feel like, and what the poke will feel like by a gentle pinch, changes the unknown to the known. Rather than using inflammatory descriptors such as "sting" or "stick," equate the puncture sensation to a mosquito bite, which is something every child can relate to. Once a child knows what to expect, a life-long fear of needles can been be averted.

It's been estimated that 10–20 percent of the population has a tendency to become needle phobic. All that is missing is a triggering event. Those who work to allay fears when they have the opportunity have the power to change lives.

(cont...)

(EMLA and other topical anesthetics cont...)

If you choose to include topical anesthetics, make sure your policy reflects the manufacturer's instructions. Most anesthetics of this type require a physician's order and must be applied up to an hour in advance. That could be a problem. If someone else applies it, for example, in a physician's office; he/she is selecting the venipuncture site for you. It may not be the same vein you'd choose.

EMLA® is a registered trademark of Abraxis Pharmaceuticals.

Did You Know...

prewarming an infant's heel or an
adult's finger prior to a skin puncture
increases the blood flow seven fold.

Heel warmers vs. warm towels or warm water gloves

Recently our phlebotomy supervisor put out a letter that only heel warmers are allowed to warm up sites for phlebotomy, and that warm towels and warm water gloves are not part of any phlebotomy procedure. Are there any specific rules saying that these alternative ways of warming up a patient are not allowed?

The best way to respond to your question is that the "rules" are whatever your employer establishes them to be in this regard. In this case, he/she is practicing good risk management.

When something other than a heel warmer is used, it opens up the potential for burning the child's foot. What feels warm to your touch might be scalding to the tender new skin of a newborn. Commercial heel warmers have a maximum temperature beyond which they do not exceed, preventing burns. According to the CLSI standards, prewarming should not exceed 42 degrees Celsius.

Heelstick, depth of puncture

Can you please tell me what the requirements are for the depth of heel-sticks on infants? Are there different depths for preemies? Also, what should I look for in a good retractable heelstick device?

The limit of puncture depth on infant heels according to CLSI is 2.0 mm. No recommendations for preemies exist. As for features, give priority to heel incision devices over heel lancet devices. Incision devices yield greater volumes of blood, require fewer repeat sticks, heal faster and are less painful to the infant.[1] Above all, prewarm all heels. It increases blood flow seven-fold.

References

1) Matthews D. Comparative studies of time requirement and repeat sticks during heelstick. *Neonatal Int Care* May/June, 1992;66–68.

2) CLSI. *Procedures and Devices for the Collection of Diagnostic Capillary Blood Specimens; Approved Standard—Sixth Edition.* CLSI document H4-A6. Wayne, PA: Clinical and Laboratory Standards Institute; 2008.

Pain management

I am always looking for ways to minimize the pain of a venipuncture, but I can't find much information on the Internet. What has been written, if anything, on the issue?

Actually, a great deal of research has been done on pain management in phlebotomy. Most of it on neonatal pain. Here's a brief rundown of what's been published:

- Topical anesthetics have been found to be effective in reducing pain[1-4], but not on newborns.[4,5]

- Lidocaine iontophoresis reduces pain responses during venipuncture.[6]

- Patients prompted to cough during needle insertion report lower pain scores than when they don't cough.[7]

- Venipunctures are less painful on newborns than heelsticks.[8,5]

- Infants being held had lower pain responses than those not held during heelsticks.[5]

- Distraction (i.e., blowing bubbles, movies, cartoons, books, parental/nurse coaching, music, counting, etc.) refocuses thinking by directing attention away from the pain.[9]

- Babies breastfed or given pacifiers, glucose, or sucrose solutions have significantly lower pain scores than those without during heelstick and venipuncture. There appears to be no optimal glucose/sucrose concentration. Glucose and sucrose are equally effective. Glucose is better than anesthetic creams in reducing pain scores. There appears to be no difference between breast-feeding and water. Babies given water and a pacifier have lower pain scores than those given neither.[5]

(cont...)

(Pain management cont...)

- Venipunctures using winged collection sets are less painful than tube-holder draws.[10]

- Watching television has been found to have an analgesic effect during venipunctures.[11]

- Finally, the *Applied Phlebotomy* textbook (available at www.phlebotomy.com) discusses four secrets to a painless puncture.

  1.) Make sure the alcohol is dry before puncturing.

  2.) Stretch the skin, making it taut.

  3.) Select a small needle (but nothing smaller than a 23-gauge).

  4.) Choose the median cubital vein whenever possible. It seems less painful to the patient, perhaps due to fewer nerve endings in the skin above this vein.

References

1) Biro P, Meier T, Cummins AS. Comparison of topical anaesthesia methods for venous cannulation in adults. *Eur J Pain* 1997;1(1):37–42.

2) Dutta A, Puri G, Wig J. Piroxicam gel, compared to EMLA cream is associated with less pain after venous cannulation in volunteers. *Can J Anaesth* 2003 Oct;50(8):775–8.

3) Rogers TL, Ostrow CL. The use of EMLA cream to decrease venipuncture pain in children. *J Pediatr Nurs* 2004 Feb;19(1):33–9.

4) Weise K, Nahta M. MLA for painful procedures in infants. *J Ped Health Care* 2005;19(1):42–7.5.

5) Franck L, Gilbert R. Reducing pain during blood sampling in infants. *Clin Evid* 2002. Jun;(7):352–66.

6) Zempsky W, Anand K, Sullivan K, Fraser D, Cucina K. Lidocaine iontophoresis for topical anesthesia before intravenous line placement in children. *J Pediatr* 1998 Jun;132(6):1061–3.

7) Usichenko T, Pavlovic D, Foellner S, Wende M. Reducing venipuncture pain by cough trick: a randomized crossover volunteer stud. *Anesth Analg* 2004;98:343–5.

8) Ogawa S, Ogihara T, Fujiwara E, Ito K, Nakana M, et al. Venepuncture is preferable to heel lance for blood sampling in term neonates. *Arch Dis Child Fetal Neonatal Ed* 2005;90(5):F432–6.

9) Cavender K, Goff M, Hollon E, Buzetta C. Parents' positioning and distracting children during venipuncture. *J Holistic Nursing* 2004;22(1):32–56.

10) Hefler L, Leodolter S, Tempfer C. To butterfly or to needle: the pilot phase. *Ann Intern Med* 2004;140(11):935–6.

11) Bellieni CV, Cordelli DM, Raffaelli M, Ricci B, Morgese G, Buonocore G. Analgesic effect of watching TV during venipuncture. *Arch Dis Child* 2006 Dec;91(12):1015–7.

Did You Know...

35% of patients feel more discomfort during a venipuncture than they expected.

Prewarming

I often hear that warming the heel increases blood flow by seven times. My employer wants us to discontinue heel warmers to save money, but if I can cite a study showing the benefit it would be helpful. Can you help?

The statement has appeared for years in the CLSI skin puncture standard.[1] The citation in the standard refers to the *Textbook of Medical Physiology*.[2] However, one study downplays the significance of heel warming and indicates further research is necessary.[3] Most experienced phlebotomists will tell you the practice is very instrumental in facilitating a good blood flow.

If prewarming were discontinued at your facility, you'd likely experience infants who require two or more puncture attempts per draw and a deterioration in specimen quality as hemolysis and tissue fluids contaminate the specimens. You would be doing your patients and laboratory a favor by strongly encouraging continuation of the prewarming policy.

References

1) CLSI. *Procedures and Devices for the Collection of Diagnostic Capillary Blood Specimens; Approved Standard—Sixth Edition*. CLSI document H4-A6. Wayne, PA: Clinical and Laboratory Standards Institute; 2008.

2) Guyton AC. *Textbook of Medical Physiology*. 10th ed. Philadelphia: W.B. Saunders Co.; 2000.

3) Barker D, Willetts B. Cappendijk V, Rutter N. Capillary blood sampling: should the heel be warmed? *Arch Dis Child Fetal Neonatal Ed* 1996;74(2):F139–40.

Skin puncture through bruised heels

Q ur neonates often have bruised heels. Does taking blood from the area of the bruise, or near the bruise, affect test results? Most of the tests we run on neonates are blood gases, electrolytes, glucose, lactate, and creatinine.

T he CLSI document H4-A6, (the skin-puncture standard) recommends avoiding a previously punctured site due to the accumulation of tissue fluid that will contaminate the specimen. Not much has been published in this area.

If you are finding that many of your neonates have bruised heels, you might want to explore how the heelsticks are being performed. The prevalence of bruised heels indicates excessive squeezing. When blood flow is so inadequate that it requires squeezing to the extent that it bruises heels, it's an indication the sites are not being prewarmed prior to puncture. As a result, not only do you get a lot of unsightly bruised heels (painful to the babies and potentially distressing to their parents), but your specimens may be hemolyzed and contaminated with tissue fluid. Both threaten the accuracy of test results. Encourage your specimen collection personnel to spend time prewarming heels more diligently with a warm compress not to exceed 42 degrees Celsius. If they spend more time prewarming, they're likely to spend less time milking blood out of heels that eventually become bruised and limit future available puncture sites.

4. Patient Identification, Vein Selection, & Site Prep

Patient Identification

Nursing-home draws

Patient identification errors in decentralized settings

Proper inpatient identification

Vein Selection

Acceptable veins in the antecubital

Ankle punctures

Abiding by the one-minute rule

Drawing from an inactive fistula

Drawing from arms with heparin locks

Drawing from edematous sites

Drawing from mastectomy patients

Draws from post-surgery mastectomy patients

Draws from the earlobe

Drawing from the underside of the arm

Draws from the same arm as ports and locks

Draws from unconventional sites

Fistulas

Foot/ankle veins

Is drawing above an IV acceptable?

Mastectomies

Mastectomy patient gives permission

Preferred vein selection

Reference for mastectomy restrictions

Scalp venipunctures

Tattooed sites

Two phlebotomists drawing one patient simultaneously

Site Prep

Cleansing puncture sites with water

Cleansing the tip of the glove

Cotton versus gauze

Correct way to wipe with alcohol

Iodine contamination

Letting alcohol air dry

Medical versus forensic blood alcohols

Patients with dirty arms

Repalpating a cleansed site

Sterile gloves and gauze for phlebotomy

Touching surfaces after donning gloves

Wiping away alcohol

Nursing-home draws

I don't understand why all long-term care residents don't have wristbands. Some patients do and some do not; most of them only have their names above their bed. It's very hard to find an employee who is not busy to help you. Once, I even had an aide bring me the wrong patient. Is there some way it could be mandatory for patients to have wrist bands?

Nursing home draws are difficult when it comes to patient identification. Such facilities strive to make their residents feel like they are in a home-like environment, which means doing away with identification bracelets. However, when a medical procedure such as a venipuncture needs to be done, the two objectives clash. Remember, the laboratory is ultimately responsible for the quality of the specimens it tests; which includes properly identifying the patients. That requires you to enforce the same policies you would in a hospital. If it's problematic to have the nurses provide proper patient identification, then you have a right to insist on arm bracelets. If neither form of identification is possible or allowed, you have a right to decline to draw their patients. It's as simple as that.

Keep in mind, even if bracelets are applied, someone still has to verbally provide the name of those patients who cannot speak their own name. This is to make sure the bracelet is on the right patient. So inconveniencing nurses is just part of the process of providing proper patient care. Just remember, patients are depending on you to be their last line of defense against specimen collection errors. That requires you to consistently apply the standards.

Patient identification errors in decentralized settings

Do you have any information on the frequency of patient identification errors in facilities that have decentralized phlebotomy versus those that have not?

Much has been written on the downside of decentralized phlebotomy, but few articles compare patient identification errors associated with decentralized phlebotomy. One, however, compares the frequency of labeling errors committed by the emergency department (ED) versus all other areas of the hospital.[1] The conclusion: the ED was ten times as likely as the rest of the hospital to submit mislabeled specimens.

Other articles discuss the frequency of rejected specimens, hemolysis, failed attempts, etc.[2-8]

References

1) Sandhaus L, Sauder K, Michelson E. Relative frequency of mislabeled laboratory samples from the emergency department (ED) compared to other hospital areas. Institute of Quality in Laboratory Medicine web site. http://cdc.confex.com/cdc/qlm2005/techprogram/paper_8547.htm. Accessed 5/16/08.

2) Nelson, K. Recentralizing phlebotomy services in the clinical lab. *Adv Med. Lab Prof* 2002;14(22):21-4.

3) Savage R (ed). Q&A. *CAP Today* 1999;13(11):97-8.

4) Southwick K. Back to the drawing board: hospitals rethink their phlebotomy staffing practices. *CAP Today* 2001;15(2):12-8.

(cont...)

(Patient identification errors in decentralized settings cont...)

5) Jones B, Calam R, Howanitz P. Chemistry specimen acceptability. *Arch Pathol Lab Med* 1997;21:19.

6) Warner, J. Recentralizing phlebotomy back to the laboratory. *Clin Lab Mgmt Rev* 2005;19(4):E3.

7) Paxton A. Stamping out specimen collection errors. *CAP Today* 1999;13(9):1–22.

8) Sauer D, McDonald C, Boshkov L. Errors in transfusion medicine. *Lab Med* 2001;32(4):205.

Did You Know...

an armband attached to the bedrail
identifies the bedrail, not the patient!

Proper inpatient identification

W hen identifying inpatients, should we ask them to state their entire name and birthday, and then check that with the labels and patient wristband? Our hospital policy states the date of birth is not necessary. Doesn't CLSI say that you need at least two identifiers?

B oth CLSI and Joint Commission (JCAHO) require two identifiers. The difference is that JCAHO allows both identifiers to come from the identification bracelet. CLSI considers that ID bracelets might be mistakenly put on the wrong patient, and requires you to not only check the bracelet, but also to ask the patient to state his/her name, address, birthdate, and/or unique identification number. The information from both sources must then be compared with the test request form. Note that the CLSI standards say "and/or." That means one or more of the items.

If the patient is unable to speak due to coma, sedation, etc., CLSI requires the collector to have a caregiver or family member identify the patient by stating the patient's name, address, birthdate, and/or unique identification number. Neither patient nor caregiver/family member can simply affirm the patient's name provided by the collector. The identifier must verbalize the name.

Acceptable veins in the antecubital

We have a question at our facility in regards to site selection for routine venipuncture. Could you tell me the sites where venipuncture is considered to be within the "standard of care," particularly in regards to cephalic, median cubital, and basilic veins? Are these veins "fair game" wherever they are located in the arm, e.g., high, low, front, back, etc.?

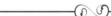

The standards require those who draw blood specimens to attempt to locate a medial or cephalic vein before drawing from the basilic vein. If either are not obvious by sight or touch, the survey should be repeated on the opposite arm if it is accessible. The median cubital vein is the vein of choice for several reasons:

- **Proximity**— a medial vein is typically the closest to the skin's surface, making it readily accessible.

- **Immobility**— a medial vein is also the most stationary of the three. This makes a successful puncture more probable.

- **Safety**— a medial vein poses the least risk of injuring underlying structures.

- **Comfort**— to the patient, a medial vein brings less discomfort when punctured. Although the vein itself has no innervation, the surface of the skin is less sensitive there than it is over the cephalic and basilic veins.

Median and cephalic veins are only the veins of choice if they are visible or palpable, and if there is a high degree of confidence that either can be accessed successfully. Selecting an indistinct medial over one of the other clearly visible or palpable veins may result in an unsuccessful attempt and subject the patient to a second puncture.

Even though collectors should select the vein that offers the highest degree of confidence, those who select the basilic vein without performing a thorough survey for safer veins are putting the patient at an increased risk of injury. That's because branches of the median antebrachial cutaneous nerve can nestle against the basilic vein. Once pierced, these nerves can send shooting pain down the length of the limb to the fingers and up to the shoulder and chest. If the injury is severe, it can be permanent. Most nerve injuries that result from punctures in the antecubital area are from errant attempts to puncture the basilic vein.

In addition to nerves, the basilic vein's close proximity to the brachial artery subjects the patient to the risk of an arterial nick and subsequent hemorrhage. Should the healthcare professional involve this artery unknowingly, the consequences to the patient can range from a barely perceptible bruising to severe hemorrhaging. Therefore, when considering punctures to the inside aspect of the antecubital area where the basilic lies, collectors should attempt to locate the brachial artery by feeling for a pulse and avoid punctures in the area if the artery lies precariously close to the basilic vein.

These risks, however, shouldn't preclude the use of this vein for the collection of blood specimens when no other vein is accessible. Often the basilic is the patient's most prominent vein. Healthcare professionals must be aware of the risk in accessing this vein, and use it only when no other vein in the antecubital area is more accessible. The CLSI standards require us to prioritize the veins for safety, and select the basilic vein only when a medial or cephalic is not accessible.

Collectors should avoid draws to the front of the wrist (palm-side) since nerves and tendons come close to the surface of the skin. Flaws in technique make this site less forgiving.

Ankle punctures

We have a physician who wants us to accept her permission to draw all her patients from the foot or ankle when necessary unless she sends a note to the contrary. I know the standards say we must obtain physician's written permission to draw from the lower extremities, but I'm leery of accepting this blanket permission unless ordered to the contrary. What should I do?

Also, if we do draw from a lower extremity, should we inform the patient to be on guard for any potential complications? Should we tell them not to put weight on the foot we drew from? ——————————— ⟨𝒢 𝒮⟩ ———————————

Injuries and complications from an ankle stick are rare, but the risks exist for phlebitis (in patients with coagulopathies) and tissue necrosis (in diabetics). Seek the physician's written permission to draw from the lower extremities of difficult-to-draw patients, and keep the record in the laboratory files. That's a necessary precaution, because we don't always know who is diabetic or who has a coagulopathy.

I'd suggest you just draft a simple form for physicians to sign indicating that ankle punctures are okay. Alternatively, you may have your medical director bring it up at the next medical staff meeting that the lab will adopt a policy allowing for ankle punctures on all patients unless the physician states otherwise. Then the burden falls upon the patient's physician to remember to make a notation on the lab order that ankle punctures should not be considered for patients they feel are at risk.

The type of "reverse permission" you are describing appears risky and may increase your liability. If the physician insists, make sure you establish her blanket permission strategy in writing. We prefer physicians approve of ankle sticks on a case-by-case basis than to have to rely on them to inform the lab when ankle sticks are not to be considered.

We have not seen recommendations on post puncture care specific to ankle sticks, so I'm assuming that the standard precautions exist as for any venipuncture. We've never seen nor heard of any weight-bearing restrictions or elevation guidelines either.

Did You Know...

up to 20 percent of the population
is predisposed to needle phobia.

Abiding by the one-minute rule

How can you stay within the one-minute tourniquet rule when finding the vein takes longer than that? Can the alcohol be removed by gauze to speed things up?

It's acceptable, even encouraged, to take your time finding a vein. But if it takes more than a minute to find, cleanse, allow alcohol to dry, and access the vein, then the tourniquet should be released. The standard says that two minutes should be allowed to pass so hemoconcentration can disperse, then retighten, relocate, re-cleanse, and stick within a minute. To make the location of the vein quicker the second time, take note of certain landmarks on the skin the first time (freckles, skin creases, hairlines, skin contours, etc.) so that when the tourniquet is applied the second time you have guideposts. Some collectors make minor indentations on the skin above a palpated vein with a ballpoint pen (cartridge retracted) when the vein is initially located (e.g., blood donor centers). Just don't take to marking the skin with ink; it's unprofessional.

Alcohol should be allowed to dry, not physically removed to expedite the draw. It's a volatile solution, so it shouldn't take more than 15 seconds to dry. You can fill that time with other preparations, so the drying phase shouldn't slow down the procedure. After the vein is located, cleanse the site. While the alcohol dries, select and assemble the needle device, apply gloves, and perform the puncture. There should be no need to remove the alcohol with gauze. By the time you've assembled your supplies and donned your gloves, it's probably dry. Besides, the drying action of alcohol kills some bacteria.

If you're teaching new students, they're less likely to move from one step to the next as quickly as you might. So they will almost always have to find the vein, release the tourniquet, assemble equipment, cleanse the site, reapply the tourniquet, anchor the vein, and insert the needle.

Drawing from an inactive fistula

I am having a difficult time with our dialysis and renal units. They are requesting that we draw from arms with dead/inactive grafts and fistulas. CLSI advises against drawing from fistulas, but does not distinguish between those that are active or inactive. Can you clarify?

Of course, drawing from active fistulas and shunts is not a good idea, but inactive fistulas should pose less of a problem. Nevertheless, there's no mention in any standards or in the literature to support this practice. It would be a good idea for your pathologist to establish a policy.

Drawing from arms with heparin locks

We have written in our procedures to treat saline/heparin locks the same as IVs when it comes to selecting a blood collection site. What that means is that, if we collect below it, we make sure it has been turned off for 3 minutes, and if we collect above, we need a signed authorization form. Many of our staff disagree with this policy because "it's only a lock," which may have had nothing running through it, ever. Any ideas of what other facilities are doing?

We know of no facility that considers heparin locks the same as active IVs when it comes to drawing blood. Nor is there anything in the literature or standards to that effect, so your staff has a point here. There is no "turning off" of a saline/hep lock, so your protocol is a bit confusing.

Drawing above an IV is done at great risk. Patients have died when results were reported on contaminated specimens drawn above IVs. CLSI cautions against it, and most textbooks agree. If you really need this option, a provision should be made that it is never to be done if the tests being drawn include analytes that were being infused. For the record, CLSI now requires specimens drawn above IVs to be labeled as such so that they won't be used for add-on tests that may not be appropriate.

Drawing from edematous sites

C an we draw blood from patients with edematous arms and hands? When all other veins are not available, I find it is possible to expose a superficial vein by applying pressure to the site for a minute or so (using the whole finger and not just the tip of the finger), and then draw from it with a butterfly set. But will the pressing down of the swollen hand/arm to expose the vein compromise test results?

T here are two issues here. Pressure on a vein may yield erroneous results if the vein is constricted for longer than one minute. After that, hemoconcentration will occur below the occlusion leading to temporary elevations of cells and high molecular weight compounds and analytes bound to protein. It's similar to the effect of leaving a tourniquet on longer than one minute. It's what we know as hemoconcentration.

But the larger issue is the compromised results that will come from drawing blood from an edematous limb. It is generally taught to avoid drawing from swollen areas as the blood flowing through them will be compromised by the excessive fluids and the abnormal physiology of the limb. The technique you described may not be a valid remedy.

Drawing from mastectomy patients

We have a woman coming in twice a year who has had a mastectomy that included removal of 18 lymph nodes. Of course, her only good vein is on the same side. She told me that her oncologist told her that it was acceptable to have blood drawn from her mastectomy side as long as a tourniquet was not used. Is it really OK to draw from that arm without using the tourniquet? If I do, what tests will have skewed results?

The rule against drawing from the same side of a prior mastectomy is hard and fast. It's not just the tourniquet that is the problem, it's any break in the skin on an affected side. That includes venipuncture or capillary puncture. Because lymph nodes have been removed, the affected side is compromised when it comes to fighting infections. The American Cancer Society's web site even cautions mastectomy patients against sewing without a thimble.

Because it is so prevalent in the literature, if a patient develops complications, the facility doesn't have much of a legal leg to stand on should she seek compensation. Even if the patient gives permission, verbal or in writing, it may not release you from liability should complications ensue. Her attorney can effectively argue that the patient was not aware of the risks involved and was not in a position to give informed consent.

However, in difficult draw situations like the one you describe, you can escape liability if you get the physician to put his/her permission in writing. The CLSI standards permit draws from the same side as a mastectomy only with physician's permission. That's your only option.

Evidence in the literature is inconclusive that test results obtained from a limb are affected by mastectomy.

Draws from post-surgery mastectomy patients

We recently had a 46-year old mastectomy patient whose surgery was six years ago. Some nodes had been removed, but she has never had any trouble or lymphedema in that arm. Is there any protocol that makes it acceptable to draw blood from the same side as a mastectomy performed many years ago?

Many patients have limitations as to their available drawing sites, but the rule against drawing from the same side of a prior mastectomy is well established in texts and in the CLSI standards. Because it is so prevalent in the literature, if a patient does develop complications, the facility doesn't have much hope of avoiding liability should she seek compensation.

However, in difficult draw situations, you can escape liability if the physician provides permission. That's your only option. Obtaining the patient's permission may not be sufficient to protect you from liability.

Draws from the earlobe

Q We have a nurse who insists on drawing blood for bedside glucoses from the earlobe. I've told her that earlobes are not recommended as a skin-puncture site by both the CLSI standard and the glucose meter's manufacturer, but she insists on the rationale before she accepts it. Why are earlobes not recommended?

A The literature is unanimous that earlobes should not be considered as acceptable skin puncture sites. However, few passages provide a reason. What's troublesome is that the employee is requesting the rationale before complying. An academic curiosity is healthy and facilitates understanding, but this curiosity sounds as if it has its origins in a rejection of authority in the form of the standards, the manufacturer's recommendations, and your facility's policy. So there are some underlying issues here that need to be addressed. Since the evidence against earlobe punctures is so well referenced, "because I said so" should be all the employee needs.

If the manufacturer of your glucose measuring system recommends against earlobe punctures, it's because the instrument was not developed or validated on samples from the earlobe. Testing earlobe samples, therefore, introduces a variable that has not been validated.

Additionally, it has been reported that test results from earlobe blood don't compare well with blood taken from the fingertip.[1] The analytes that vary include hemoglobin (significantly increased), hematocrit (significantly increased), and pH (significantly decreased).

Here's what some of the most reliable authorities in the industry had to say about your predicament:

- Terry Jo Gile, aka "The Safety Lady™": My OSHA resource suggests that earlobe punctures may put the healthcare worker at risk should the sharp penetrate the thin flesh of an earlobe.

- Dan Baer, columnist for MLO magazine: In one study, blood circulation in earlobes was shown to be slow, perhaps due to vasoconstriction from the cold. If there is reduced flow of blood, the glucose metabolism would be different from that in capillary blood in more rapidly flowing capillaries.

- Roger Calam, MD, Lab Administrator, St. John Hospital in Detroit and CLSI standards advisor: There would probably be significant apprehension for some patients if a phlebotomist was seen approaching the side of their head with a puncturing device. Children could be very disturbed by this collection. An obvious obstacle to this collection is the ever-increasing incidence of earrings, even pediatric patients increasingly presenting this way. The CLSI rationale as I remember it for not recommending this procedure was because it is so uncommon and therefore should not be encouraged. If a diabetic wishes to pursue this technique and there are no adverse results, then more power to them. But in a clinical setting, it's not recommended.

Reference

1) Young D. *Effects of Preanalytical Variables on Clinical Laboratory Tests*, AACC Press. Washington, DC. 1997.

Drawing from the underside of the arm

I have a person who requests to be drawn from the backside of the lower arm, with the needle pointing in the direction from the elbow to the wrist. This seems like an awkward vein to draw and an awkward direction in which to access it. Should I comply? ————————⟨ᵷ⟩⟨ᵹ⟩————

You have to be very cautious about letting the patient select the site for you. It's nice to be able to honor a patient's wishes, but ultimately it's not the patient's choice. When drawing outside of the recognized and acceptable veins (i.e., the antecubital, back of the hand, and side of the wrist), one may have a difficult time defending one's choice should an injury occur. One should never draw anywhere without knowing the anatomy of the area and the risks involved. Just because it's the patient's preference, it will not immunize you against liability should an injury occur. All veins are not fair game.

Even if the vein the patient selected was an acceptable vein, it may not be a good idea for you to comply. For example, if the patient insists you draw from the basilic vein (the one in close proximity to the nerves and brachial artery), but a safer medial or cephalic vein is available, you should tactfully decline.

According to CLSI, you must survey both arms, if accessible, for the presence of a medial or cephalic vein before selecting the basilic vein. Since the medial and cephalic veins are least likely to put the patient at risk of a nerve injury or arterial nick, they must be considered before drawing from the riskier basilic... even if the basilic is the patient's preference. You simply can't let the patient's preference take precedence over the standards.

If the patient becomes insistent you draw from a basilic when safer veins are available, you should contact your supervisor before taking it upon yourself to operate beneath the standard of care. Should there be an injury, the patient's attorney can successfully argue that the patient wasn't knowledgeable enough about the risks involved in drawing from the basilic vein to be given the authority to select the site of the puncture. As a venipuncture specialist, you are expected to have the expertise to make a better judgment of the venipuncture site than the patient.

Did You Know...

nerves can pass over the basilic vein
as well as beneath and along side of it.

Draws from the same arm as ports and locks

We are in a clinic setting where patients come in for outpatient blood draws, and are not equipped or trained to draw from saline locks or ports. We need to know the proper procedure for drawing blood from these patients. Of course the obvious solution is to use the other arm, but if that arm cannot be used, what site should be used for the draw? Is it permissible to draw blood from below the port site? If so, should a tourniquet be applied?

It's always acceptable to draw below a port or lock. The proper procedure is to apply the tourniquet below the device, puncture below that, and document that it was drawn below a port. As long as nothing is being infused into the site, you should be able to draw above a port or lock, as well. But you may or may not always have that information. If you know it, document the time and solution of the last infusion/injection to allow for proper interpretation of the results.

Draws from unconventional sites

I am corporate legal counsel for a healthcare system in the Midwest. One of our hospitals has an acutely ill patient who has been hospitalized more than 100 times. She has no viable veins in her extremities from which to draw blood. Her physician feels it should be the phlebotomist's responsibility to draw blood from a vein in the breast or in the stomach. The laboratory director feels this is not within the scope of practice of a phlebotomist. Is this true? Is there is any resource that specifically states in writing what the scope of practice for a phlebotomist actually is?

The phlebotomy profession is largely unregulated. As such, it has no official "scope of practice" except in California. However, this is not so much a scope-of-practice issue as it is a standard-of-care issue.

The laboratory director is correct that draws from such unorthodox sites are beneath the standard of care for phlebotomy. The acceptable sites for venipuncture are the bend of the arm (antecubital area), back of the hand, and thumb-side of the wrist. Feet and ankles are acceptable only with physician's permission. Should complications arise from draws to any other area, the risk of liability increases dramatically. The physician may feel all veins are fair game, but that's contrary to the standards.

If the nurse or physician wants to draw blood outside of the acceptable areas, they do so at their own risk. Keep in mind that most nurses and physicians get little or no phlebotomy instruction in their professional training, hence the more cavalier approach to the procedure. Laboratory professionals, on the other hand, receive comprehensive training, and their professional opinions should carry the greater weight.

Fistulas

Q Is there any information available regarding phlebotomy through a fistula?

A lthough CLSI doesn't give a rationale, their standard states not to use an arm with a fistula for blood draws routinely. The risk is in starting an infection that renders the fistula unusable for dialysis, which would be a serious complication for the patient. If you have a patient with a fistula, and draws elsewhere are difficult, get the physician's permission, preferably in writing.

Foot/ankle veins

I need to find information in regards to phlebotomy of the foot. All I am finding so far is information on heelsticks, not venipunctures. What's out there?

Generally, foot and ankle punctures should not be performed without physician's written permission. The risks are that if the patient is diabetic, he/she may develop tissue necrosis due to a diabetic's inability to heal in the lower extremities. If the patient has a clotting disorder, feet or ankle punctures can lead to phlebitis and other clotting complications. Since the physician is the best to assess the risk to the patient, the CLSI standards state that he/she give permission first. Getting permission in writing is good risk management should anything happen.

Is drawing above an IV acceptable?

Can you tell me what the protocol is for collecting specimens below an IV? Is there any situation when a specimen collected above IV is acceptable for analysis?

CLSI recommends draws to the same arm as fluids are being infused should be avoided whenever possible.[1] When not possible, the recommendation is to draw below the IV by shutting it off for two minutes (or having the nurse do so if IV management is not in your scope of practice), tightening the tourniquet below the IV, collecting the specimen below the tourniquet, and documenting that the specimen was drawn from an arm being infused. Some texts add the step of discarding the first 5 cc as an additional precaution.

As for drawing blood above an IV, studies show that accurate lab results can be obtained as long as the IV is shut off for two to three minutes and the analytes being tested were not being infused (e.g., glucose, sodium, chloride, potassium, antibiotics, etc.). The infusing fluids must be documented. From a practical standpoint, this is a very risky practice for the facility to permit. The CLSI venipuncture standard leaves it up to the facility to establish its own policy.

The risk is greatest in facilities that have deployed blood collection responsibilities to some units where non-laboratory personnel are allowed to draw specimens as well as phlebotomists. For example, a nurse may observe a phlebotomist—who is aware of the limitations drawing above an IV for labs that don't include what's being infused—and conclude that it must be okay to draw above an IV in all situations. That's when the exceptions fall to the wayside, and before you know it the lab is receiving specimens contaminated with IV fluids.

Another risk is that tests could be added on to stored blood originally drawn above an IV. Even though the original sample may have been drawn for tests that didn't include any of the analytes being infused, the add-on tests could. CLSI requires specimens drawn above or below an IV to be labeled as such.[1] For these reasons, allowing blood to be drawn above an IV is a perilous policy.

References

1) CLSI. *Procedures for the Collection of Diagnostic Blood Specimens by Venipuncture; Approved Standard—Sixth Edition.* CLSI document H3-A6. Wayne, PA: Clinical and Laboratory Standards Institute; 2007.

2) Read D, Viera H, Arkin C. Effect of drawing blood specimens proximal to an in-place but discontinued intravenous solution. *Am J Clin Pathol* 1988;90(6)702–706.

3) Savage R, ed. Q&A column. *CAP Today* 2002:16(4):102–103.

Did You Know...

George Washington died after his physician performed a large-volume therapeutic phlebotomy as treatment for a cold, essentially bleeding him to death.

Mastectomies

Our hospital is seeking research evidence that supports or refutes doing venipunctures in the arm on the mastectomy side. We have found an expert opinion that states it is permissible to do venipunctures on the affected side because 1.) the risk of lymphedema is less now since fewer lymph nodes are removed and 2.) when sterile technique is used for the venipuncture.

We have found equal opinions to the contrary due to the risk of infection or precipitation of lymphedema. Could you direct us to solid evidence in the literature so we can settle this issue once and for all?

You are correct that mastectomies are done with less removal of lymph nodes today than in the past. But the problem is that not all mastectomies are done that way, depending on the surgeon and the extent of the metastasis. This begs the question: how is the person who draws from a mastectomy patient supposed to know the extent of the mastectomy? Since some mastectomies may still be radical, it's not prudent for the phlebotomist to assume lymph node preservation on every patient.

The reference you're looking for is the standard for venipunctures published by the Clinical and Laboratory Standards Institute (CLSI), document H3. It states physician's permission must be obtained before drawing on the same side of the mastectomy. It makes no exception for the extent of lymph node removal or time since the mastectomy. Not even a bilateral mastectomy precludes the necessity for physician's permission. No one but the physician is in a better position to know the extent of lymph node removal. As such, he/she needs to be consulted if your facility is to operate within the standard of care.

Given the weight of the standards in legal proceedings, I doubt the lack of additional articles matter should the patient drawn on the same side of a prior mastectomy sue for pain and suffering. Nevertheless, the following journal articles relate to complications after mastectomy that can be attributed to venipuncture and skin puncture on the affected side:

1) Savage R. (ed.) Q&A. *CAP Today* 1995;9(5):63–64.

2) Simon M, Cody R. Cellulitis after axillary lymph node dissection for carcinoma of the breast. *Am J Med* 1992;93:543–548.

3) Getz D. The primary, secondary and tertiary nursing interventions of lymphedema. *Cancer Nurs* 1985;8:177–187.

4) Brennan MJ, Weitz J. Lymphedema 30 years after radical mastectomy. *Am J Phys Med Rehabil* 1992 Feb;71(1):12–4.

A copy of the venipuncture standard stating this requirement is available for a fee as a download or printed booklet from the Center for Phlebotomy Education's web site www.phlebotomy.com/Downloads.html or directly from the Clinical and Laboratory Standards Institute at www.clsi.org.

Did You Know...

in most states you need a license to cut someone's hair, but not if you want to insert a needle into their vein to draw blood.

Mastectomy patient gives permission

One of our patients wanted to give me permission to draw from the same side as her mastectomy, which she had 30 years ago. I refused, and I think it made her kind of mad. Was I right?

Even if the patient says it's okay, don't expect her permission to hold up in court should she develop complications and sue for pain and suffering. The patient's attorney could effectively argue that she wasn't aware of the complications that could ensue from granting permission, and didn't have a full knowledge of the consequences. The argument will likely continue that it is the healthcare professional who should be versed in the risks of drawing from the affected side. A patient's permission to deviate from the standard of care just doesn't hold up in legal proceedings very well.

So, yes, you were correct to refuse to draw from that side without the physician providing the permission. If she left in anger, you might consider explaining the rationale better, stating that facility policy doesn't permit you to draw from the arm, even with her permission.

Preferred vein selection

I am a medical assisting student and we are using a book instructs to always use the cephalic and basilic veins in the antecubital area. It said nothing about the median cubital. I had been taught that it isn't wise to use the basilic because it is too close to the brachial artery and the median nerve. What's the current thinking?

You are right about the erroneous vein selection priority that the book advocates, and about the reasons the basilic should be attempted only after ruling out the cephalic and median veins. This proves not all texts are well researched on phlebotomy, especially those that serve non-laboratory professions.

Reference for mastectomy restrictions

Do you have any other sources besides the CLSI standard that restricts venipunctures on mastectomy patients?

Here's what's in the literature on collections from mastectomy patients that does not cite the CLSI standard, but supports it:

- *Illustrated Manual of Nursing Practice*. Springhouse Corp. Page 1333. 1994.

- *The Lippincott Manual of Nursing Practice*. Lippincott-Raven Publishers. Philadelphia, PA. 1996.

- Q&A. *Laboratory Medicine* 1999;30(2):93.

- Strasinger S, DiLorenzo M. *The Phlebotomy Workbook, 2nd edition*. FA Davis Company. Philadelphia, PA. 2003.

- McCall R, Tankersley C. *Phlebotomy Essentials. 3rd edition*. Lippincott Williams & Wilkins. Philadelphia, PA. 2003.

All these sources caution against drawing blood from the same side as a prior mastectomy (in addition to the American Cancer Society's web site[1]) and serve as a basis for the CLSI restriction.

Reference

1) Lymphedema: what every woman with breast cancer should know. http://www.cancer.org/docroot/mit/content/mit_7_2x_lymphedema_and_breast_cancer.asp. Accessed 5/16/08.

Scalp venipunctures

I s there any literature on the safety of collecting blood samples from scalp veins in small children? It appears to be a practice sometimes used by physicians, but we are not sure if any laboratories perform the procedure on a consistent basis. Any light you could shed on this for us would be greatly appreciated.

S calp veins are a legitimate site for venipuncture on newborns and infants, but it's rarely performed. Neither laboratory-based phlebotomists nor techs are typically trained to access scalp veins. Instructional information on performing scalp vein punctures can be found in Garza and Becan-McBride's *Phlebotomy Handbook*. It's available on amazon.com and other traditional outlets.

Tattooed sites

I've got a friend with tattoos. He said most phlebotomists usually look at the tattoo (thin lines, over veins, but not covering veins completely), then go to his other arm. What's your take on drawing through tattoos? Not new tattoos, but old, well established ones?

Some texts advise against drawing from tattooed areas on the grounds that dyes may interfere with testing, they are more prone to infection, or have impaired circulation. This is largely perceptual and without supporting evidence in the literature. CLSI makes no mention of restrictions on such sites, new or old.

Two phlebotomists drawing one patient simultaneously

What do you think about two phlebotomists drawing blood cultures on a patient from opposite arms at the same time? I was taught never to do this, but at my new job they do it all the time. I thought that if both arms were tied off, the patient could pass out. What's the real truth on this method of drawing blood?

Teaming up for two sets of blood cultures at the same time sounds a bit odd. The results would not likely be compromised, but it's quirky and seems like a poor use of personnel. If both arms are available, one phlebotomist could just as easily draw from each arm consecutively as two can concurrently. The only benefit in teaming up is in saving time, but we're only talking about ten minutes or less. So it's a little puzzling why two would be assigned to do what one can.

Because there's no support for it in the literature, I'd discourage the practice. It doubles the volume of blood being constricted from circulating, which may not be a good idea in acutely or chronically ill patients.

Cleansing puncture sites with water

t the clinic I work, we recently had a patient who said he was allergic to alcohol and iodine when he came in for a lab blood draw. He stated that where he used to get his blood drawn, the phlebotomist would clean the site with sterile water. We cleansed his arm with soap and water and then drew the blood. Is this ok?

terile water is fine. Soap and sterile water is better. Remember, a venipuncture is not considered a sterile procedure (unless it's for culture). So I don't think you should have any trouble with cleansing this patient's site as you described.

Cleansing the tip of the glove

Can you repalpate the site after cleansing the tip of your glove?

There is a real temptation to reestablish contact with the vein after the site has been prepped to make exactly sure where to insert the needle, but it isn't appropriate. Gloved fingers are rarely decontaminated as scrupulously as the patient's skin. There are other ways to retain vein location after initial palpation. Instead, repalpate above and below the intended puncture site, but not the site itself, Also, take note of certain landmarks on the skin when you locate the vein the first time (freckles, skin creases, skin contours, etc.). They can serve as guideposts so that when you reapply the tourniquet, the second attempt to locate the vein doesn't take as long. Some people make an indentation on the skin where the vein was found with a ballpoint pen (cartridge retracted) or fingernail. Making a mark with ink, though, is unprofessional. But cleansing a gloved finger and repalpating the site of needle insertion is not acceptable.

Cotton versus gauze

We are using cotton balls at our facility instead of gauze. In the *Applied Phlebotomy Video Series*, gauze is recommended. Is this a mandatory requirement, or just a recommendation?

The CLSI standards caution against using cotton for the same reasons mentioned in the video: when the cotton is lifted from the site, the fibers of the cotton, which may have become embedded into the fragile fibrin plug, can pull the plug from the puncture, reopening the wound. However, it's okay to use cotton to apply alcohol for the purpose of site preparation. But gauze is the recommended pad for applying post-venipuncture and post-skin puncture pressure.

Correct way to wipe with alcohol

What's the right way to cleanse a site for routine labs? I have always wiped the alcohol in concentric circles, and continue to teach that method. However, some of my coworkers at this hospital went to an in-service regarding site preparation, and were told that concentric circles were unacceptable and that the new method is one swipe down with an alcohol pad followed immediately by one swipe with a gauze pad.

You are correct to question the source of such information. It sounds like another example of someone trying to reinvent the procedure. The CLSI venipuncture standard still says you should cleanse the site using concentric circles of increasing diameter starting from the anticipated needle insertion point to the outside, a few inches in diameter. It also says that it should be allowed to air dry.

Alcohol has an antiseptic effect when allowed to air dry. Not that phlebotomy is a sterile procedure, but there's no harm in letting alcohol kill microbes by letting it air dry.

Iodine contamination

I have a question from the ER nurses concerning IV draws and iodine/povidone interference. The concern is how much is the iodine interfering with the potassium, phosphorous, and uric acid when it's left on the skin after site cleansing. What would happen if they wiped off the iodine with alcohol before the draw and let it dry? Does a chlorhexidine scrub affect chemistries in the same way?

One article states that potassium, uric acid, and phosphorous are all increased when a skin puncture site is prepped with iodine, but doesn't say by how much nor cite a reference.[1] Nor does it suggest the same contamination occurs when a venipuncture is performed. However, co-authors of a letter to the editor of *Clinical Chemistry* report their own internal study that quantitates the effect. They report that potassium increases about 25% while uric acid decreases 11%.[2] Unfortunately, the reference is quite dated and includes blood drawn by venipuncture from only one patient. Bicarbonate and chloride have been reported to increased when measured on Kodak Ektachem systems (now Ortho/J&J Vitros), but this comes from a "personal communication" written in 1994 and cited in a compendium of preanalytical effects, not a study. Since the personal communication is not published, it's impossible to know if the author experienced the contamination during a venipuncture or skin puncture.[3]

You could avoid this contamination by removing the iodine with an alcohol prep as you suggested. Just make sure the alcohol is dried before puncturing. If not, the residual alcohol could hemolyze red cells. We know of no study that has measured analyte interference from chlorhexidine preps.

References

1) Becan-McBride, K. (ed) Preanalytical phase and important requisite of laboratory testing. *Advance for Med. Lab. Prof* Sept. 28,1998:12–17.

2) Van Steirteghem A, Young D. Povidone-iodone ("Betadine") disinfectant as a source of error. [Letter] *Clin Chem* 1977:23(8):1512

3) Young D. *Effects of Preanalytical Variables on Clinical Laboratory Tests*. AACC Press. Washington, DC. 1997.

Did You Know...

Iodine in tincture form has been found to be
more effective in reducing contamination
rates than iodine in povidone form in facilities
that have deployed phlebotomy responsibilities
to a multi-skilled workforce.

Letting alcohol air dry

Please help me with my question about gauze. Can you wipe the alcohol off the venipuncture site with a piece of gauze before you put the needle in the arm, or are you just supposed to let the alcohol air dry? What does CLSI say about this?

CLSI says we should allow the area to air dry in order to prevent hemolysis of the specimen and to keep the patient from experiencing a burning sensation during needle insertion. It's not bactericidal, but some organisms are killed during the drying process. So wiping it away prematurely prevents that important action.

There's a reason the standard states "air dry" instead of "dry the site" or "allow the site to dry." That's because we don't want people blowing on it or waving air over it, both processes introduce bacteria onto the site. It's all about good hygienic practices.

Medical versus forensic blood alcohols

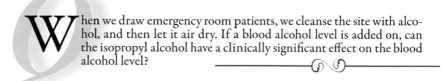

When we draw emergency room patients, we cleanse the site with alcohol, and then let it air dry. If a blood alcohol level is added on, can the isopropyl alcohol have a clinically significant effect on the blood alcohol level?

For most testing methodologies, isopropyl alcohol does not interfere with ethyl alcohol determinations. So if the physician orders an ETOH level for medical purposes, prepping the site with isopropyl alcohol shouldn't be a concern.

If the medical records are then subpoenaed to prosecute the patient, convincing a jury that the results are valid may be difficult. If it is brought to light that the site was prepped with isopropyl alcohol, it may create a reasonable doubt. To a jury without knowledge of clinical chemistry, convincing them the results were not affected will be a tough sell.

Your best approach is to treat all blood alcohol requests as if they had forensic potential, and prep the patient without compounds or soaps that contain alcohol of any kind. If you don't have access to non-alcohol compounds, the use of water and gauze with modest friction may be an option. Above all, follow your facility's protocol. (Venipuncture is not considered a sterile procedure unless you are drawing blood cultures.) If a forensic alcohol is added to tests collected using conventional site prep solutions, a repeat venipuncture would yield more bulletproof results.

Patients with dirty arms

From time to time I will have a person who is so filthy that I want to just stick their whole arm in the sink and wash it with soap and water before drawing his/her blood. One is a regular, and I swear he must spread diesel fuel and coal dust on his arms before he comes in each time. The last time I had to do a venipuncture on him, I used five alcohol swabs to clean the site. Please tell me what to do when he comes back again.

This is an interesting and delicate question. From a customer service standpoint, sending the patient home to wash up would be bad form. Most patients wouldn't want to be embarrassed by having to be so thoroughly scrubbed when they come in either. It seems avoiding embarrassment is clearly not a motivator with this patient, so you'll have to find something else. I would recommend asking him to wash his arm thoroughly before he comes in next time, explaining that if he does, you can get him in and out faster and he can get on with his day. Giving him some benefit in the process is likely to be the only way to motivate him to wash first.

If that doesn't work, you'll just have to accommodate his poor personal hygiene and have soap, water, and a washcloth available. It may not be a bad idea to cleanse his site with iodine or chlorhexidine to sterilize it. If a thorough washing doesn't get him clean enough, at least the dirt remaining would be sterilized.

Repalpating a cleansed site

I understand that when drawing blood cultures, a sterile environment is created and that, once prepped, the site cannot be re-palpated prior to venipuncture. Does that hold true for routine venipunctures as well or can I repalpate a site cleansed with only alcohol?

Sites prepped with alcohol should really remain untouched. Even though alcohol doesn't sterilize it, it's good infection control to avoid repalpating the site. Since over 100,000 patients die each year from nosocomial infections, 75% of them preventable, I would discourage the practice.[1] According to the CLSI standard, the site should be cleansed again if a difficult venipuncture leads the collector to touch the site after initial cleansing.

Reference

1) Berens, M. Tribune investigation: unhealthy hospitals. *Chicago Tribune.* July 21, 2002. http://www.ahrp.org/infomail/0702/23.php. Accessed 5/16/08.

Sterile gloves and gauze for phlebotomy

We have been approached by a physician asking why normal venipunctures are not performed as a sterile procedure using sterile gloves and gauze. Do you have any background or sources that I might use to address this with the physician who is promoting that all venipunctures be performed as a sterile procedure?

Being a minimally invasive procedure, sterile gloves are no more necessary than they are for administering an injection. If contaminating the puncture site were a problem under the current standards, we would certainly be hearing about it from the infection control folks. But we aren't because it isn't.

Request the physician provide proof, rather than opinion, that phlebotomy should be a sterile procedure. No such proof exits unless blood cultures are ordered. The lack of evidence is why sterility is not required by standards organizations.

Touching surfaces after donning gloves

I occasionally get complaints from nursing and outpatient draws that when my techs don the gloves, they still open drawers and touch tubes and other nonsterile supplies. They complain that we are not following sterile procedures when drawing blood. How should we tactfully share with them what donning the gloves is all about?

If donning gloves was to maintain a sterile field, nurses would don gloves when they administer an IM injection. But they don't because the risk of infection is infinitesimally small.

Phlebotomy is not a sterile procedure. But it never hurts to minimize the gloves' exposure to contaminated surfaces before coming in contact with the patient. It's good infection control. The more surfaces their gloves touch, the more bacteria the compromised patient will be subjected to. Since over 100,000 patients die each year in the US from nosocomial infections, you should make sure your staff is aware of the threat contaminated gloves bring to the patient, and minimize contact with contaminated surfaces after donning gloves.

Wiping away alcohol

The way we prep a site for venipuncture is to wipe with the alcohol pad in a circular motion. We then use unsterile gauze to wipe excess alcohol so that it doesn't sting during needle insertion. Should I be allowing the site to air-dry versus wiping with gauze? If we choose to wipe with gauze, must it be sterile? Is it acceptable to use non-sterile gauze at any time during the phlebotomy?

Non-sterile gauze is acceptable for phlebotomy, but the alcohol should be allowed to dry on its own.

Venipunctures are not a sterile procedure (except when drawing blood cultures), so non-sterile gauze is acceptable. However, it's not considered appropriate to wipe off the alcohol. You should let it air dry instead. The drying process does have some bactericidal effects, so the site will be more decontaminated than if you wipe away wet alcohol.

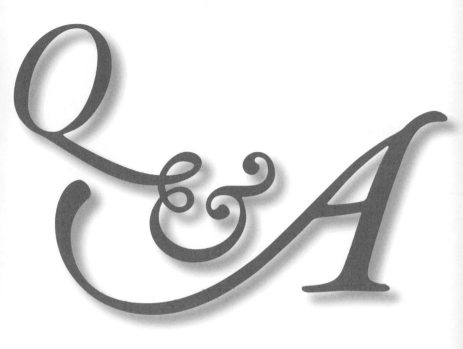

5. Tourniquets & Butterflies

Tourniquets

Tourniquet hygiene
Tourniquet time
Tourniquets, drawing without

Butterflies

Butterflies and needlestick rates
Butterfly overuse
Butterfly requests by patients
Butterfly use
Using butterflies on hand veins

Tourniquet hygiene

Currently, we use one tourniquet on multiple patients. What is the standard practice? Should we be using a tourniquet only once per patient and then discarding it?

There are no guidelines or standards that say you must use a tourniquet once and throw it away. However, many hospitals have this policy. It's more of an infection control issue to prevent nosocomial infections.

The CLSI standards don't say anything about tourniquet hygiene; published studies are inconclusive. Without a clear guidance from the literature, consider including the following in your protocol:

- Discard tourniquets that are visibly soiled or contaminated with blood.

- Whenever possible, tighten tourniquets around the sleeve of the patient's shirt or garment to prevent pinching and skin contact.

- Discard tourniquets that fall on the floor.

- Use a new tourniquet on patients in isolation and discard after use.

Some facilities issue a tourniquet to their patients upon admission, which remains with them throughout their hospitalization. It would be a good idea to consult with your facility's infection control officer in developing your new tourniquet policy.

Tourniquet time

I work in a clinical research facility. A recent question came up about the length of time the tourniquet may safely be applied to a person's arm and the regulation governing this. I have read that two minutes is recommended. However, we have timed the procedure and found that, to obtain the number of tubes requested for this study, it needs to stay on up to four minutes. Where might I find this issue addressed?

Four minutes sounds like a long time to obtain specimens. When the tourniquet is left on longer than one minute, significant changes take place in the blood trapped in the veins below it. The effect is known as hemoconcentration, and it starts altering test results within one minute of application. Once hemoconcentration occurs, you get a temporary elevation in cellular components of the blood below the constriction as well as protein-bound and high molecular weight analytes.

Drawing the specimen when the blood is hemoconcentrated can lead to inaccurate results and medical errors when the physician acts upon them. This is stated in most text books and originates in the CLSI standard H3. The standard is available from the Center for Phlebotomy Education's web site (www.phlebotomy.com) or from CLSI directly at www.clsi.org.

To minimize hemoconcentration, the tourniquet can be released as soon as the vein is accessed, as long as it is felt it will not threaten the success of the puncture. If it takes longer than one minute to find and access the vein, the tourniquet should be released for two minutes so that the blood can return to its basal state. Once found, you can relocate the vein quickly after the tourniquet is reapplied by making a mental note of where the vein lies in relation to certain skin markers like creases, freckles, and surface contour.

Tourniquets, drawing without

I have a phlebotomist who is very experienced and does not use a tourniquet. This creates problems with the patients because the next time they come in, they request no tourniquet. How do other institutions respond to these special requests?

Your "experienced" phlebotomist is operating beneath the standard of care. The standards require a tourniquet for finding a vein (unless its use alters the analyte being tested, such as lactate).

It's my guess she/he doesn't know that the nerve most commonly injured during venipuncture is near the basilic vein. Without a tourniquet, how can one possibly find another vein, one with a lower risk, and effectively reduce the risk of nerve injury? All who draw blood specimens should prioritize veins for safety.

When patients start requesting your staff to operate beneath the standard of care, you have a problem. Your ability to manage risk deteriorates precipitously. Your experienced phlebotomist needs information on nerve damage and arterial risks. I suggest the "Avoiding Phlebotomy-Related Lawsuits" DVD, and the "Blood Collection Sites and Precautions" wall atlas, both available from the Center for Phlebotomy Education (www.phlebotomy.com).

Butterflies and needlestick rates

I recognize that the only acceptable needlestick injury rate is 0%, but the management and safety groups here are looking for statistics to try to support decreasing the number of butterfly collections. Can you tell me what an "acceptable" injury rate is, or maybe you have some information on the decrease of injuries after OSHA legislated safety products. Also, are you familiar with any information on the number of butterfly collections vs. straight needle (tube holder) collections used in different facilities?

After safety legislation was enacted in the US in 2001, the frequency of sharps injuries went down from 38 per year for every 100 beds in 2000 to 22 two years later. (Source: International Healthcare Worker Safety Center).

As recently reported in the journal, *Infection Control and Hospital Epidemiology*, one facility experienced a 93% reduction in accidental needlesticks after converting to safety needles.[1] As for needlesticks from butterflies alone, one statistic says butterflies are responsible for 32 percent of all accidental needlesticks to phlebotomists.[2] For the general healthcare professional, a CDC report in 1997 said that 83 percent of percutaneous injuries sustained with safety needles were caused by butterfly needles (pre-safety legislation).[3] Of those, 61% occurred before activation, 15% during activation and 20% occurred because the device wasn't activated.

Post-legislation data shows a decrease in all exposures by 51% including a 70% decrease in phlebotomy needle exposures and a 55 percent decrease in butterfly needle exposures.[4] We have seen no data on the frequency of butterfly usage.

References

1) Valls V, Lozano M, Yánez R, Martínez M, Pascual F, et al. Use of safety devices and the prevention of percutaneous injuries among healthcare workers. *Infect Control Hosp Epidemiol* 2007 Dec;28(12):1352–60.

2) Jagger J. (1994) Risky procedure, risky devices, risky job. *Adv Exp Prev* 1994;(1):4–9.

3) Evaluation of Safety Devices for Preventing Percutaneous Injuries Among Health-Care Workers During Phlebotomy Procedures -- Minneapolis-St. Paul, New York City, and San Francisco, 1993–1995. Centers for Disease Control and Prevention. *MMWR* 1997;46(2).

4) Pyrek K. Study shows needlestick injuries on the gradual decline. *Inf Ctrl Today* 2003;7(6):39.

Did You Know...

61% of all accidental needlesticks sustained during phlebotomy procedures occur within seconds of when the needle is removed from the patient's arm.

Butterfly overuse

What are your thoughts on the high usage of tube holders with butterflies by specimen collection personnel who are required to draw blood? I keep thinking that if you have to use the butterfly, it's because the vein is too small/fragile for a tube-holder draw, so why would you put a vacuum at the end of the butterfly?

Butterfly over-usage is a problem everywhere. They should be reserved for fragile veins and used primarily with a syringe. If a tube holder can be used, there's no need for the butterfly in most cases. It's up to your facility to enforce conservative use of these devices. If your staff overuses them, it's probably for the same reason everyone else does: they're very maneuverable, patients request them, and they require less of a steady hand to maintain placement during the draw. However, they are also associated with a high rate of accidental needlesticks (EPINet data).

Perhaps you might recruit your infection control nurse to launch a campaign on appropriate use of butterflies. You will still have to stock them for those difficult geriatrics and pediatrics, but that means they'll still be available for overuse. If you could get the point across about butterflies and accidental needlesticks (no pun intended), you might be able to induce a behavioral change.

Butterfly requests by patients

I am a phlebotomy supervisor for a military hospital. I remember reading a *Phlebotomy Today* "Tip of the Month" on patients who want to tell me where to stick them and that I have to use a butterfly. I am very respectful when it comes to patients who have had a hard time having their blood drawn, but I need to put my foot down somewhere. How do I respond to patient requests that I'm not comfortable with?

Demanding patients can be very frustrating. While it's important to have good customer service skills, one has to balance patient satisfaction with your own safety. If you are uncomfortable using a butterfly set when circumstances don't require them, tactfully resist by telling patients that you're more likely to get accidentally stuck with a butterfly than with a regular needle. (Studies have shown that thirty-two percent of all accidental needle-sticks to phlebotomists come from butterfly needles.) Explain that you're much more comfortable and successful using a regular needle. Most patients won't push you to work outside your comfort zone. If push comes to shove, you may opt to have someone else draw the patient. If you're uncomfortable with the increased risk, you should not be forced to compromise your safety.

As for requests to use small needles, they're a lot easier to honor.

Butterfly use

I am a stat phlebotomist for a local hospital who routinely needs to stick patients in the geriatric population. What risks are associated with using butterfly needles? I would speculate that I use them on 90% of the patients I draw. Any suggestions or ideas why this would be a problem?

Studies have shown that 32% of all accidental needlesticks phlebotomists sustain are from butterfly needles. Granted, this study involved non-safety butterflies, but EPINet data suggests the emergence of safety needles on the market has not reduced the frequency of accidental needlesticks from butterlfy sets to the same degree as other blood collection devices. Because of this, most organizations advocate minimizing butterfly use whenever possible.

Geriatric patients often require butterfly needles, but we suggest evaluating each patient regardless of age and make the safest decision you can. If you can use a tube holder, do so. Just make sure you avoid using butterfly sets exclusively on all geriatric patients just because they're geriatric.

Using butterflies on hand veins

On hand veins, I find that I am much more successful using butterfly sets with tube holders attached than with just using a tube holder with a safety needle attached. As long as I don't let go of the wings, I am usually successful. I think it has to do with the fact that I use glass tubes, not plastic. Glass tubes have less vacuum. Is there anything wrong with my technique?

On hand veins and small veins, the full force of the vacuum applied to the inside of a vein can collapse it onto the bevel, restricting blood flow. It sounds like that is not your experience, but many collectors prefer to use a syringe with either a safety needle or butterfly set attached, so that they can control the pressure applied within the vein.

Historically, butterfly sets have been associated with a disproportionately high accidental needlestick rate for phlebotomists (EPINet data). Combined with their increased cost, there are more than enough reasons to wean yourself off of them as much as possible.

As for plastic tubes having less vacuum than glass, that's debatable. The same amount surely must be necessary to fill the tube regardless of what the tube is made of. Regardless, you really should consider switching to plastic tubes. OSHA mandates plastic wherever possible to prevent broken glass exposures. There are plastic counterparts for every blood collection tube, including blood culture bottles.

6. Order of Draw & Discard Tubes

Order of Draw

Order of draw: black-stoppered tubes

Order of draw: capillary blood gases

Order of draw: citrate carryover

Order of draw: tissue thromboplastin

Order of draw for ACD tubes

Order of draw with clot activators

Order of draw with syringes

Revised order of draw for emergencies

Serum tubes in the order of draw

Trace element tubes in the order of draw

Discard Tubes

Discard tube

Discard volume for heparinized line draws

Discard volumes for vascular-access draws (VADs)

Discard volumes when drawing above an IV

Order of draw: black-stoppered tubes

What would be the correct placement in the order of draw of Ves-tec tubes for the Mini-ves Sed rate system? The anticoagulant is 0.109 mol/L sodium citrate. Should it be drawn after the light blue top?

Also, some of the phlebotomists remove the tube from its plastic case before inserting into the tube holder. Since the test records the change in opacity of the blood, would there be a problem with touching the reading part of the tube since it is acting like a cuvette?

While it is true that coag tubes containing sodium citrate should come first in the order of draw, the placement of non-coag tubes with the same additive, such as those you are wondering about, is less critical. You can safely draw black-stoppered tubes containing sodium citrate after the coag tube or as the last tube. Any additive that carries over into it should not affect the sed rate, not even a clot activator, which will be overwhelmed by the anticoagulant.

More than likely, the manufacturer of the sed rate tubes you are using does not recommend removing them from the plastic tube for filling. Your concerns about the tube being misread are valid.

Order of draw: capillary blood gases

Do you know if there is a recommended order of draw when performing heelsticks on children, particularly on our preemies? We've been told that the hematology specimens should be collected first because of the risk of clots beginning to form if the collection becomes lengthy. But it's also recommended that the capillary blood gas be obtained before the baby begins to scream and cry too much as that activity will affect the blood gas results. Are you aware of a particular protocol for these draws?

You are correct on both accounts. Once the capillary beds are arterialized and the puncture is performed, the blood emerging becomes increasingly more venous and less arterial. So if the ABG is delayed in the order of draw, the results obtained will be increasingly inaccurate.

Likewise, if the collection of the CBC is delayed, there is an increased likelihood of erroneous cell counts due to platelet clumping. When properly arterialized, the ABG should be collected relatively quickly. The potential for platelets to clump should be minimal. If you want to assure both tests are as accurate as possible, you might consider performing separate punctures.

Order of draw: citrate carryover

When a sodium citrate (blue top) tube is drawn before a serum tube, as recommended in the CLSI order of draw, isn't there a potential for some of the sodium citrate additive to carry over into the serum tube, potentially affecting chemistry tests, like sodium? Proper technique requires us to make sure that the tube is oriented with the tube stopper uppermost, keeping the anticoagulant from coming in contact with the interior needle, but this isn't always practical. How can we prevent sodium citrate carryover from affecting the results obtained from the serum tube that follows?

If all tubes were filled from bottom to top as you described and the interior needle never came in contact with the blood: anticoagulant mixture, an order of draw wouldn't be necessary. But we know that it's not possible to orient all draws with the tube in this manner. That's why an order of draw is necessary. With the order of draw maintained, any additive carryover is irrelevant.

CLSI establishes its standards, including the order of draw, on published articles and studies. There has been no evidence in the literature that indicates sodium citrate, if it does carry over, affects the results of the tests conducted on the next tube. Without any evidence, the effect remains theoretical.

Order of draw: tissue thromboplastin

It is my understanding CLSI changed the order of draw in 2003 so that it is now:

1.) blood culture tubes;

2.) blue tops;

3.) red tops;

4.) green tops;

5.) purple tops;

6.) gray tops.

It is also my understanding that if a blue top is the only tube to be drawn, it no longer needs a waste tube unless it is being drawn with a butterfly. This is contrary to several things I had read in the past (i.e., that the clot-activator tubes should not be drawn before anticoagulant tubes because of possible contamination, and also that tissue thromboplastin in the needle could interfere with a blue top drawn by itself.) Can you help clarify this for me please?

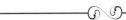

No study has ever proven that tissue thromboplastin interferes with coagulation studies. It's always been speculation until the late 1990s when studies proved that drawing a discard tube before the citrate tube made no difference in protime and aPTT results. Therefore, CLSI discontinued their recommendation for a discard tube in 1998 when drawing a protime or aPTT.[1,2]

However, studies have not been conducted on any affect of tissue thromboplastin on special factor assays. CLSI guidelines and standards, therefore, state that evidence of tissue thromboplastin contamination is consequential at best, and that facilities should establish their own policy in regards to special factor assays.

There is certainly no harm done when drawing a discard tube, it's just not necessary when testing for protimes and aPTTs. Of course, discard tubes are still recommended when drawing with a butterfly set and the blue top is the first or only tube drawn. This is to prevent short sampling when the air in the tubing enters the citrate tube. The discard tube need not be filled, but only applied long enough to prime the line of the winged collection set. The discard tube can be another citrate tube or a plain, non-additive tube. As far as the clot activator contaminating an anticoagulant tube, there is no evidence in the literature that this occurs or that it affects results.

References

1) CLSI. *Collection, Transport, and Processing of Blood Specimens for Testing Plasma-Based Coagulation Assays and Molecular Hemostasis Assays; Approved Guideline—Fourth Edition.* CLSI document H21-A5. Wayne, PA: Clinical and Laboratory Standards Institute; 2008.

2) CLSI. *Procedures for the Collection of Diagnostic Blood Specimens by Venipuncture; Approved Standard—Sixth Edition.* CLSI document H3-A6. Wayne, PA: Clinical and Laboratory Standards Institute; 2007.

Did You Know...

the first evidence that collection tube additives carry over and can corrupt the results obtained in the next tube appeared in the literature in 1977.

Order of draw for ACD tubes

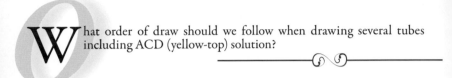

What order of draw should we follow when drawing several tubes including ACD (yellow-top) solution?

There are just far too many different types of tubes to have an order of draw that includes them all. That's why you'll never see an order of draw that includes more than the most commonly used tubes. What this means is that the collector has to know the additive and how it can affect the tube to follow should it carry over during needle transfer. Also, it's important for the collector to know what the tube in question is being used for, and to determine if the tube before it has an additive that will interfere with the test should it carry over. It would be nice if it were simpler, but something as complex as preanalytical physiology can only be simplified so far.

To answer your question, it depends on what the yellow tops are being used for. If they are being used for blood culture collections, they would go first, of course. If they are used for leukocyte testing or other esoteric tests, put them at the very end, which would be immediately following the EDTA tube. Since EDTA chelates calcium, additive carryover shouldn't affect CD4 or other leukocyte analyses.

Order of draw with syringes

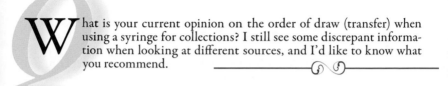

W hat is your current opinion on the order of draw (transfer) when using a syringe for collections? I still see some discrepant information when looking at different sources, and I'd like to know what you recommend.

T here's no shortage of discrepancy on the order of draw. CLSI has never recommended a separate order for syringes. It started to appear in the literature in the 1980s, but in 1998, CLSI put the issue to rest in H3-A4 by saying a separate order of draw is not necessary.

Some textbook authors were, and still are, of the opinion that clotting in the barrel of the syringe during the draw necessitates an evacuation of the blood into anticoagulated tubes first, with the non-additive red-top tubes last. But such speculation is without merit; no studies support the accelerated clotting theory. In fact, since most syringes are plastic, the coagulation cascade doesn't proceed as rapidly as it does within glass tubes, glass being a clot activator itself.

Bottom line: tubes filled by syringes should be in the same order as when filled by tube holder.

Revised order of draw for emergencies

Our written venipuncture procedure states the order of draw as: citrate, SST/clot, heparin, EDTA. Our Emergency Preparedness Plan currently states that when a trauma alert (i.e., disaster) is called, the order of draw changes to: EDTA (for BB/hematology purposes), citrate, heparin, and then the clot tube. I understand the need for BB/hematology to take priority in this kind of situation, but how does this revised order square with the risk of anticoagulant cross-contamination?

There's no support in the literature for such a modification. It sounds as if the person behind this revision lacks an understanding of the rationale behind the order of draw. It's difficult to understand why an emergency would demand a revised order of draw. Will there be someone standing by during every venipuncture to rush each tube to the laboratory as soon as it's filled? You should vigorously discourage attempts to reinvent such a well-established procedure.

Serum tubes in the order of draw

Why would a red-stopper tube without additives now be drawn after a blue-stopper tube? Isn't there the possibility for additive carryover? We still draw some red-stopper glass tubes without additive for some special send out tests. ⎯⎯⎯⎯⎯⎯⎯⎯⎯

There's nothing wrong with drawing a red-stopper tube before a citrate tube as long as the red stopper tube does not contain a clot activator. With the prevalence of plastic serum tubes on the market, CLSI moved glass red tops behind the citrate tube (where clot-activator tubes were positioned) in 2003 because there is no evidence that sodium citrate carries over and affects serum studies.

CLSI bases its documents on scientific evidence. We know that EDTA carries over based on published studies, but there has never been a study that showed citrate carries over and affects results. Therefore, rather than to have two orders of draw, one for glass and one for plastic, the current order of draw works for both and keeps it simple.

Trace element tubes in the order of draw

Our laboratory has been discussing the order of draw, and there is one tube that we are uncertain about: the trace element tube (royal blue stopper). It contains sodium heparin and we use it for copper and zinc testing. Is this collected in the same position as any other heparin tube (i.e., after the serum tube but before the EDTA), or is it collected first because the glass or plastic in other tubes may contain trace elements that could carry over and contaminate it?

Also, do trace element tubes need to be collected by syringe?

Trace element tubes have to be collected in a manner that prevents contaminants in the stoppers themselves from accumulating in the needle that pierces each one in a multiple-tube collection, and then carrying them over into the specimen to be tested.

- If a needle/tube holder assembly is used for the collection, it's best to perform a separate venipuncture for the trace element tube. Putting the trace element tube first in the order of draw is not an acceptable alternative, since its additive could carry over into the next tube.

- If you are drawing into a syringe, fill the other tubes in the proper order of draw, then change the safety transfer device so a fresh one is used to puncture the trace element stopper.

- If you are drawing blood cultures, avoid drawing the trace element tube first, as it could transfer bacteria from the nonsterile trace element stopper into the blood culture bottles.

- If you are drawing a citrate tube (for coags) after the trace element tube, some of the sodium heparin could carry over and affect the coagulation studies. When drawing with a tube holder, a separate venipuncture would be required.

When a trace element is ordered, save the patient a stick and yourself the time by drawing with a syringe and changing safety transfer devices before filling the trace element tube.

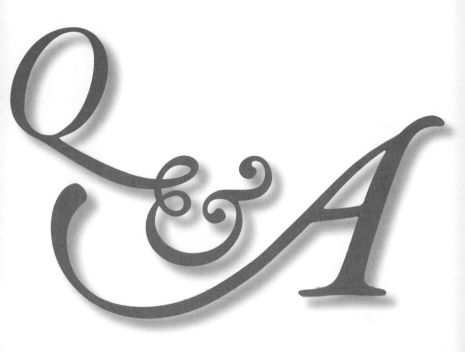

Discard tube

Q There's a lot of confusion at our facility about when we need to draw a discard tube. Can you clear this up for us?

A The practice of withdrawing and discarding a portion of blood before filling a coag (blue top) tube is old school. Truth be told, tissue thromboplastin, long thought to accumulate in the needle during the venipuncture, has never been proven to alter coag results. In fact, many studies have shown that if the citrate tube is the first tube drawn, protimes and aPTTs are not affected.

The recommendation for a discard tube was dropped in 1998 when the CLSI, the agency that establishes the standards for blood collection procedures, determined that there was insufficient evidence to support the practice. However, they still recommend it under two circumstances: 1) whenever specific factor assays are drawn such as Factor VIII; and 2) if you are drawing through a butterfly set. No studies have been attempted to determine whether or not tissue thromboplastin affects special factor assays. So CLSI suggests facilities establish their own protocol for such tests.

When using butterfly sets, you should apply a discard tube long enough to evacuate the air from the tubing so that the patient's tube filled isn't underfilled. Then apply the tube to be tested. Blue-top tubes must be filled at least 90% of their volume in order for the coag studies to be accurate. There isn't much leeway.

When employed, a discard tube can be another coag tube or a plain, non-additive tube.

Discard volume for heparinized line draws

W hen drawing from lines in which heparin is being infused, our policy is to flush with saline, draw off 5 mL of waste, then collect the specimen for testing. The nurses consistently pull off lesser volumes. I would really like us to be consistent with the standards. What do they say?

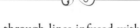

C LSI recommends we avoid drawing through lines infused with heparin if at all possible. If not possible to avoid, the line should be flushed with 5 mL of saline followed by the withdrawal and discarding of twice the dead-space volume of the vascular-access device (VAD) for noncoagulation testing, and six times the dead-space volume, for coagulation tests.

These standards and guidelines provide a descriptive, step-by-step for the collection of diagnostic blood specimens by venipuncture. They serve as the basis for any laboratory procedure, including phlebotomy, and apply to all healthcare personnel. Just keep in mind that the standards do not change just because a nurse is performing the procedure. It's still a laboratory procedure and the laboratory is responsible for the quality of the specimens it tests. CLSI standard H3 is available for a fee as an immediate download or bound publication from the Center for Phlebotomy Education's web site (www.phlebotomy. com/Downloads.html) or directly from the Clinical and Laboratory Standards Institute at www.clsi.org. For additional information, please refer to:

1) CLSI. *Collection, Transport, and Processing of Blood Specimens for Testing Plasma-Based Coagulation Assays and Molecular Hemostasis Assays; Approved Guideline—Fourth Edition.* CLSI document H21-A5. Wayne, PA: Clinical and Laboratory Standards Institute; 2008.

2) CLSI. *Procedures for the Collection of Diagnostic Blood Specimens by Venipuncture; Approved Standard—Sixth Edition.* CLSI document H3-A6. Wayne, PA: Clinical and Laboratory Standards Institute; 2007.

Discard volumes for vascular-access draws (VADs)

Can you give a nurse-friendly definition of a vascular-access device's "dead space?" In addition, what would you consider the lesser of two evils for clearing the dead-space: drawing a red-top sprayed with clot activator or drawing an extra coag tube (if that is the first tube to be collected)? The problem is that we just switched to a low volume coag tube (2.7 mL) and that's not enough to clear the dead-space. ———————

The dead-space volume is that volume of fluid the line holds between where a syringe would be attached to withdraw the blood out and the aperture that opens up into the bloodstream.

According to the CLSI standards, the discard volume should be twice the dead-space volume of the catheter for all labs except coags, which require 6 times the dead-space volume.[1,2] Drawing off 5 mL protects against dead-space volumes of 0.8 cc. Drawing off 10 mL protects against dead-space volumes of 1.65 cc. However, those who draw blood from vascular-access devices don't always know the device's dead-space volume, and researching it would take too much valuable time. You can either do a survey of the lines in use in your facility to see what the maximum dead-space volume is, and establish a policy based on your findings, or you can routinely discard 5 mL from all VADs. That's why the standard also says 5 cc should be adequate for all draws.

You are correct that a low-volume coag tube wouldn't be enough to clear the recommended dead-space volume. But there's a bigger problem here than just obtaining an adequate discard volume.

You should discontinue the use of a tube holder attached to your VAD if you want to prevent hemolysis. Studies show that tube holders attached to VADs result in specimen hemolysis up to six times more frequently than when a syringe is attached to the device to withdraw the specimen.[3,4]

Nevertheless, if you're drawing directly into tubes using a tube holder attached to the VAD, and a coag tube is required, it's not advisable to draw into a clot activator tube as a discard tube since it is conceivable that some of the activator can carry over into the coag tube and corrupt the results. Instead, use two low-volume coag tubes or a plain non-additive tube, but not a clot activator tube. Clot activators are considered additive tubes, too.

References

1) CLSI. *Collection, Transport, and Processing of Blood Specimens for Testing Plasma-Based Coagulation Assays and Molecular Hemostasis Assays; Approved Guideline—Fourth Edition.* CLSI document H21-A5. Wayne, PA: Clinical and Laboratory Standards Institute; 2008.

2) CLSI. *Procedures for the Collection of Diagnostic Blood Specimens by Venipuncture; Approved Standard—Sixth Edition.* CLSI document H3-A6. Wayne, PA: Clinical and Laboratory Standards Institute; 2007.

3) Grant M. The effect of blood drawing techniques and equipment on the hemolysis of ED laboratory blood samples. *J Emerg Nurs.* 2003;29(2):116–21.

4) Stankovic A, Smith S. Elevated serum potassium values: the role of Preanalytic variables. *Am J Clin Pathol* 2004;121(Suppl1):S105–Sl12 5105.

Did You Know...

a study on blood cultures drawn on emergency room pediatric patients found that draws from the antecubital fossa are least likely to be contaminated.

Discard volumes when drawing above an IV

I am writing to confirm whether or not it is appropriate to draw 5–7 mLs of blood as a discard tube when drawing above an IV that has been shut off for at least 5 minutes. According to other publications and our own laboratory manual, it is supposed to be done. When I reminded everyone in a staff meeting, our lab manager and some of my employees challenged me. Can you help me form an authoritative answer for them?

The real underlying question here is why your facility allows blood to be drawn above an IV at all. Studies show that certain analytes can be falsely elevated when drawn above active IVs that have been temporarily shut off.[1,2] It's not that there is a dilution factor, but that if the IV contained analytes that are being tested, they can lead to falsely elevated results. According to the CLSI standards, facilities should establish their own policies after taking this potential into consideration.

Theoretically, you can successfully draw above a temporarily discontinued IV as long as you are not drawing for analytes that were being infused. The problem with this policy, though, is twofold:

1.) What if you draw above a temporarily discontinued IV for analytes not being infused, and then the physician adds on tests later for analytes that happened to be infused at the time of the draw? For example, a metabolic profile is added to a specimen previously drawn above a temporarily discontinued IV for a liver panel. The lab tech pulls the specimen without knowing it was drawn above an IV, reports out an elevated potassium that prompts the physician to react in ways that can be potentially tragic to the patient. Even though CLSI's latest venipuncture standard requires the specimen to be labeled as such, not all facilities have caught on to the requirement.

2.) What if you work in a facility in which specimens are drawn by laboratory-based phlebotomists and nurses? Let's say the nurse in the intensive care unit couldn't get a blood sample, so she called for the laboratory to send up a phlebotomist. The phlebotomist has the nurse shut off the IV, waits two minutes (the recommended time to wait after shutting off an IV), then draws the tests because she knows that the tests ordered do not include any analytes that were being infused. The nurse watches the phlebotomist draw above the IV and assumes it's okay to do so with all patients, not knowing the exceptions. The next week she draws a metabolic panel above a temporarily discontinued IV thinking it must be okay since she watched the lab phlebotomist do it last week. The next thing you know, an erroneous test results prompts the physician to react inappropriately with potentially tragic results. It's an all-around risky policy.

But if you must draw above an IV, the recommendation is to discard up to 5 mL before collecting the specimen to be tested. CLSI requires specimens drawn above or below an IV to be labeled as such.[3]

References

1) Read D, Viera H, Arkin C. Effect of drawing blood specimens proximal to an in-place but discontinued intravenous solution. *Am J Clin Pathol* 1988;90(6)702–706.

2) Savage R. (ed.) Q&A. *CAP Today* 2002;16(4).102–3.

3) CLSI. *Procedures for the Collection of Diagnostic Blood Specimens by Venipuncture; Approved Standard—Sixth Edition.* CLSI document H3-A6. Wayne, PA: Clinical and Laboratory Standards Institute; 2007.

7. Hemolysis & Potassium Issues

Hemolysis

ER blood culture contamination & hemolysis

Hemolysis and 25-gauge needles

Hemolysis and butterfly sets

Hemolysis and IV draws

Hemolysis, causes

Hemolysis chart

Hemolysis in the ED

Frequency of hemolysis

Potassium Issues

Elevated potassiums from fist pumping

Elevated potassiums that don't repeat

High potassiums in lithium heparin tube

ER blood culture contamination & hemolysis

Our ER has been drawing blood for about three years now, and we continue to have trouble with blood culture contamination and hemolysis. I educate and train their techs who will be drawing blood, but the problem seems more with nursing. How do you handle education with emergency room staff?

Every ER shares your frustration. A study reported in the *Journal of Emergency Nursing* describes a similar issue at a hospital like yours where the authors, all nurses, investigated the lab's claim that they were hemolyzing specimens during collection in the ER. The nurses didn't believe they were responsible and conducted their own study to prove it. The results showed the lab was right: their draws were more hemolyzed than laboratory phlebotomists' draws. Here's the reference:

- Kennedy C, Angermuller S, King, R, Noviello S, Walker J, et al. A comparison of hemolysis rates using intravenous catheters versus venipuncture tubes for obtaining blood samples. *J Emer Nurs* 1996;22(6):566–569.

Don't be overly critical of the nurses, however. In the ER, everything has to happen quickly, and they give a priority to expediency. That's the driving force behind draws during an IV start. Unfortunately, such expediency is at odds with a good specimen, which is the laboratory's priority. Understanding the difference in priorities is key to working together. Try explaining how draws during IV starts can be more detrimental to the patient than beneficial, especially when the diagnosis and treatment is delayed because of a hemolyzed specimen that has to be recollected by venipuncture.

As for blood culture contamination, the same force is at work. Reinforce that whether the antiseptic is iodine or chlorhexidine, it requires at least 30 seconds of contact in order to decontaminate the site. Expediency here cuts that time short and you end up with skin flora growing inside the culture bottles presenting a misperception of the patient's condition.

Hemolysis and 25-gauge needles

I have always been taught that a 25-gauge needle will hemolyze a specimen and affect patient results adversely. But my staff argues that if this is true, why do manufacturers make them? I don't have an answer for that. I hate being the mean old phlebotomy supervisor and tell my staff they can't use them just because I said so. How do I answer their challenge?

Your staff's argument that the availability of 25-gauge needles justifies their use is irrational. Just because 18-gauge needles are available, does that mean that they can use them, too? Of course not.

You are exactly right about 25-gauge needles causing hemolysis. Tell your staff 25-gauge butterflies are available, but they have limitations, they often compromise specimens, and should only be used when it clear that no other needle will work. For example, venipuncture on infants or geriatrics where veins are so small or fragile, that a 23-gauge needle will blow the vein. By no means should they be considered for routine draws. Take a stand and stick to it. It's up to you to define the boundaries; expect for them to be challenged.

Hemolysis and butterfly sets

I am an IV therapy educator. We have a physician who is requesting we only use 21-gauge needles when we draw blood because 23-gauge butterflies cause hemolysis. Most of our patients have chronically poor venous status, which does not allow for use of such a larger-bore needle. We have no supportive documentation that indicates any needle-specific hemolysis. Do you?

This claim is likely based on mere speculation rather than solid evidence. No evidence exists in the literature supporting the claim that 23-gauge needles hemolyze specimens any more than 21-gauge needles, or that butterfly needles hemolyze specimens more than any other blood collection needle. It's doubtful the physician making this request can provide any supportive evidence, either.

Hemolysis and IV draws

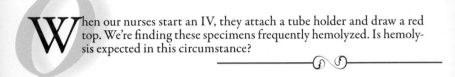

Q When our nurses start an IV, they attach a tube holder and draw a red top. We're finding these specimens frequently hemolyzed. Is hemolysis expected in this circumstance?

A Vascular access devices are notorious for hemolyzing red blood cells. Every facility that draws blood during an IV start has a hemolysis problem. Guaranteed. The best way to prevent hemolysis is to avoid using an IV for the purpose of drawing blood. Statistics show they're 10 times more likely to hemolyze a specimen than drawing by venipuncture.

Even though IV cannulas may be of the same gauge as a blood collection needle, they're not made for drawing blood. Therefore, they have a design that doesn't consider the fragility of red blood cells. We know that the interior of a blood collection needle is smooth and without interruption, but assuming the same for any other vascular-access device is overly presumptuous.

Hemolysis, causes

We are experiencing an abnormal number of hemolyzed samples. These samples are being sent to our core lab and, upon analysis, the appropriate disclaimers are placed on the results. When I drill down on this issue I've discovered that there are three different types of blood drawing going on:

1.) med techs using 21g & 23g needles;

2.) med techs who will only use a 23g or 25g butterfly, and;

3.) RNs who usually draw the blood samples when they are inserting the IV catheter. They all seem to have an equal number of hemolyzed samples.

I was taught that the use of butterflies should only be considered when the first attempt with the tube holder assembly fails and a second stick is required. As for the use of IV catheters, I've never experienced a problem with drawing blood from these devices in the past. Can you give me some insider hints relating to this problem?

Your experience with IV catheters is unique. Most facilities struggle with hemolysis of specimens drawn through vascular-access devices, whether drawn at the time of the insertion of the IV or after. It is considered an inherent problem with such draws, and facilities with hemolysis problems are well advised to minimize the frequency of line draws.

However, your problem doesn't seem to be a function of personnel or devices. Other causes of hemolysis include:

- vigorous mixing of the specimen after collection;
- using too small of a needle;
- improper needle placement in the vein;
- red cell fragility;

(cont...)

(Hemolysis, causes cont...)

- wrong blood:anticoagulant ratio (i.e., underfilled tubes);
- excessive plunger pressure on syringe draws.

Discontinue the use of 25-gauge needles wherever possible. This size may be contributing to your hemolysis rate. Oncology patients are difficult to draw, but reserving this needle only for extreme circumstances—and then only with very delicate pulling pressure on the syringe—might bring your rate down.

It could also be possible that hemolysis is occurring during specimen storage or transport. Based on your question, it sounds like the oncology clinic performs their own draws, then sends the specimens to you. Could it be that they are spinning the tubes in the office at an excessive speed? Rimming their clots and re-spinning? Are the specimens exposed to excessive temperatures? Are they being transported through a pneumatic tube system? Investigate these potential contributors. It's a frustrating problem, but there's an answer in there somewhere.

Did You Know...

in Uganda, where 25% of patients have HIV, 55% of all healthcare workers sustain two accidental needlesticks per year. (Source: Bandolier Library.)

Hemolysis chart

D o you know of any source of information that defines the levels of hemolysis? We are searching for information that would help us standardize what "trace, 1+, 2+, 3+, 4+" actually means relative to hemolysis. Are there any color comparison charts available that grade hemolysis?

T here are two places in the literature where the hemolysis chart you're looking for can be found: the March, 2003 issue of *Transfusion* (Volume 43, page 297) and the November, 2006 issue of *MLO* (*Medical Laboratory Observer*) (Volume 38, No. 11, page 26).

The *Transfusion* chart shows eight levels of hemolysis and indicates the quantity of red cells ruptured in mLs corresponding to each level. The *MLO* chart also shows eight levels of hemolysis, but gives the amount of hemoglobin in each in mg/dL instead. Some manufacturers of chemistry analyzers also provide similar charts.

Hemolysis in the ED

We have been working on a chronic hemolysis problem in our ER. We've explored many options, including the various connecting devices in use in that department. Lately the ER nurses have started to put the blame on the lab. Although we doubted that possibility, we've been investigating ourselves in all fairness. We discovered that there are conflicting recommendations about how blood should be stored and transported. The CLSI guideline H18 mentions keeping tubes in an upright position. Is there any evidence supporting this?

Tube orientation is not likely contributing to your hemolysis rate. Your story mirrors almost exactly a study reported in the *Journal of Emergency Nursing* where the authors, all nurses, investigated the lab's claim that they were hemolyzing specimens during collection in the ER. The nurses didn't believe they were responsible and conducted their own study to prove it. But what they proved is that their draws actually were more hemolyzed than those drawn by laboratory phlebotomists. Here's the reference:

- Kennedy C, Angermuller S, King, R, Noviello S, Walker J, et al. A comparison of hemolysis rates using intravenous catheters versus venipuncture tubes for obtaining blood samples. *J Emer Nurs* 1996;22(6):566–569.

More than likely, your nurses are hemolyzing specimens drawn during IV starts. If you can discourage this practice, your hemolysis rates would plummet. Vascular-access devices simply aren't designed for blood to be withdrawn but for fluids to be infused. So when used for a purpose for which they're not intended, you're going to get the results you're getting. The problem is worse when hemolysis is not detected and the compromised results are released, as for CBCs and H&Hs released by the hematology department. Unless the specimen is centrifuged—which CBC specimens aren't—there's no way to tell that it's hemolyzed.

If you run into resistance, try having them use syringes instead of tube holders so that the pressure at the tip of the line is minimal and less likely to rupture red cells, or to limit draws only to larger gauge cannulas (such as 18 gauge or larger).

Frequency of hemolysis

We are struggling to get our hemolysis rate down. It would be helpful to know what the rate of hemolysis is industry wide as a percentage of all specimens drawn. That way, I can tell how serious our problem really is. Does such a benchmark exist?

At least four studies have measured the frequency of hemolysis in emergency department (ED) draws, but only one on overall draws. Generally, the range of hemolysis during venipuncture in the ED is 0.3 percent to 3.8 percent. The summaries of the articles and citations are below.

- The hemolysis rate in blood drawn during ED venipunctures was found to be 3.8%.[1]

- Hemolysis in ED samples drawn by venipuncture was <1%.[2]

- 0.3% of samples drawn in the ED by venipuncture were hemolyzed.[3]

- Specimens drawn by laboratory-based phlebotomists showed a 1.6% hemolysis rate.[4]

- 3.3 percent of all specimens collected for clinical testing are hemolyzed.[5]

References:

1) Kennedy C, Angermuller S, King R, Noviello S, Walker J, et al. A comparison of hemolysis rates using intravenous catheters versus venipuncture tubes for obtaining blood samples. *J Emerg Nurs* 1996;22(6):566–569.

2) Grant M. The effect of blood drawing techniques and equipment on the hemolysis of ED laboratory blood samples. *J Emerg Nurs* 2003;29(2):116–21.

(cont...)

(Frequency of hemolysis cont...)

3) Lowe G, Stike R, Pollack M, Bosley J, O'Brien P, et al. Nursing blood specimen collection techniques and hemolysis rates in an emergency department: analysis of venipuncture versus intravenous catheter collection techniques. *J Emerg Nurs* 2008;34(1):26–32.

4) Burns E, Yoshikawa N. Hemolysis in serum samples drawn by emergency department personnel versus laboratory phlebotomists. *Lab Med* 2002;5(33):378–80.

5) Jones BA, Calam RR, Howanitz PJ. Chemistry specimen acceptability. A College of American Pathologists Q-Probes study of 453 laboratories. *Arch Pathol Lab Med* 1997;121:L19–26.

Did You Know...

incisions from heel incision devices heal
faster than punctures from lancet devices.

Elevated potassiums from fist pumping

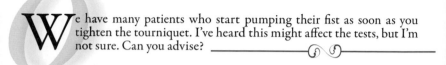

We have many patients who start pumping their fist as soon as you tighten the tourniquet. I've heard this might affect the tests, but I'm not sure. Can you advise?

Fist-pumping increases levels of potassium, lactic acid, and ionized calcium while it decreases the blood's pH. Its affect has many citations in the literature including:

- Dale J. Preanalytic variables in laboratory testing. *Lab Med* 1998;29:540–545.

- Renow BW, McDonald JM, Ladenson JH. The effects of stasis with and without exercise on free calcium, various cations and related parameters. *Clin Chim Acta* 1980;103:91–100.

- Narayanan S. The preanalytic phase: an important component of laboratory testing. *Am J Clin Pathol* 2000;113:429–452.

- Baer D, Ernst D, Willeford S, Gambino R. Investigating elevated potassium values. *MLO* 2006;38(11):24–31.

- Young D. *Effects of Preanalytical Variables on Clinical Laboratory Tests*. AACC Press. Washington, DC. 1997.

You should discourage the practice.

Elevated potassiums that don't repeat

I n the past three months, we have reported elevated (crisis) potassium levels to physicians ten times. The physicians send the patients back for a redraw only to find that the level is normal. In the beginning, we looked at the obvious, i.e., temperature, centrifugation, length of tourniquet application, and the pumping of a patient's fist during the draw. We changed policies in order to assure that all specimens within our realm of control are spun within one hour after collection, and still we are having this problem occur. Do you have any suggestions of how to handle this? Is there anything we could be missing?

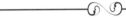

S purious, unexplained potassium results haunt every laboratory sooner or later. Investigating them requires a comprehensive review of a multitude of preanalytical and patient variables. Here's a rundown of factors that contribute to spurious potassium levels, including those items you already investigated:

1.) Make sure your staff is adhering to the proper order of draw. If someone is putting the EDTA tube before the tube to be tested for electrolytes, you can get a substantial carryover effect. The same thing happens when someone pours off some of the blood from an EDTA tube into a tube to be tested for potassium if the draw failed to yield enough blood for both. It happens.

2.) Make sure the questionable draws are not from above an IV.

3.) Make sure specimens are not refrigerated before centrifugation.

4.) Make sure specimens are not recentrifuged a second time.

5.) Gross hemolysis can increase a potassium level by 1.5 mEq/L or more.

6.) Make sure your staff isn't leaving the tourniquet on longer than one minute, forcing hemoconcentration below the constriction.

7.) Make sure your patients aren't allowed to pump their fists.

8.) Make sure you are properly flushing and discarding before drawing from vascular-access devices.

9.) Make sure your specimens are centrifuged within two hours of collection.

10.) Make sure your staff isn't rimming clots, which hemolyzes red cells.

11.) Make sure you consider the contribution that elevated white blood cells and platelets of patients with myeloproliferative diseases make to the measured potassium.

12.) Make sure you're not considering serum and plasma potassium to be equivalent (serum potassium is 0.4 mEq/L higher on average).

13.) Make sure your elevated levels are not due to being drawn during the insertion of benzalkonium IV catheters.

14.) Make sure the tube's gel barrier is intact and doesn't allow contact between serum/plasma and cells.

Bibliography

1) Dale, J. Preanalytic variables in laboratory testing. *Lab Med* 1998;29:540–545.

2) Renow B, McDonald J, Ladenson J. The efforts of stasis with and without exercise on free calcium, various cations and related parameters. *Clin Chim Acta* 1980;103:91–100.

3) Narayanan S. The preanalytic phase an important component of laboratory testing. *Am J Clin Pathol* 2000;113:429–452.

4) Baer D, Ernst D, Willeford S, Gambino R. Investigating elevated potassium values. *MLO* 2006;38(11):24–31.

5) Young D. *Effects of Preanalytical Variables on Clinical Laboratory Tests.* AACC Press. Washington, DC. 1997.

6) Handy B, Yu S. Evaluation of potassium values in a cancer patient population. *Lab Medicine* 2005;36(2):95–7.

7) Sevastos N, Theodossiades G, Savvas S, Tsilidis K, et al. Pseudohyperkalemia in patients with increased cellular components of blood. *Am J Med Sci* 2006;331(1):17–21.

8) Ernst D. Case Study: investigating spurious potassium results. *ASCLS Today* 2002;16(8):8–9.

High potassiums in lithium heparin tube

We have periodic problems with high potassium levels on lithium heparin plasma specimens received from our outreach clinics. The specimens are spun down and arrive on ice three to twelve hours after collection. Many of them are cooler than room temp when tested. What could be causing our problem?

There are a lot of processes in play here that could be affecting your potassium levels. You didn't mention if your heparin tubes have a gel separator or not, so let's assume they don't for the sake of a complete answer. If that assumption is correct, one of the factors is that the plasma is remaining in contact with the cells. When kept in contact, the potassium moves from the cells (which have 23 times as much potassium than the plasma) into the plasma.

The other obvious issue here is that the specimens are transported on ice. Refrigeration accelerates the process of potassium leaching from the cells into the plasma. According to CLSI, separation from the cells should occur within two hours of collection if testing for glucose, potassium, and a slew of other tests. Refer to CLSI document H18, *Procedures for the Handling and Processing of Blood Specimens*.

If your heparin tubes have a gel separator, then neither plasma/cell contact nor the cold transport temperature is the issue, provided centrifugation was adequate and the specimens were not refrigerated prior to centrifugation. Make sure you are centrifuging them at the appropriate rcf according to the tube manufacturer's recommendation. If the centrifuge is a fixed-angle style, the gel barrier may be thick on one side and perilously thin on the other. Such centrifuges are notorious for providing inadequate separation of plasma and cells. The problem may not go away until and unless a swivel-head centrifuge is put in place that spins the tubes at a 90-degree angle to the rotor.

Alternatively, you might ask your tube manufacturer if they can provide you with a double-gel tube for centrfuging in fixed-angle centrifuges. At least in the short-term it may be a more affordable solution than replacing centrifuges.

Finally, make sure you're not comparing plasma potassium levels to serum potassium levels and expecting them to be equivalent. As blood clots, the platelets release potassium. By nature, serum potassium levels will be higher than plasma potassium levels by as much as 0.4 mmol/L. Much of this information is scattered about the literature in multiple publications, but a good summary article appeared in the November, 2006 issue of MLO. (See Baer reference below.)

Bibliography

1) Baer D, Ernst D, Willeford S, Gambino R. Investigating elevated potassium values. *MLO* 2006;38(11):24–31.

2) Young D. *Effects of Preanalytical Variables on Clinical Laboratory Tests*. AACC Press. Washington, DC. 1997.

3) NCCLS. *Procedures for the handling and processing of blood specimens; Approved Standard—Third Edition*. CLSI document H18-A3. Wayne, PA: Clinical and Laboratory Standards Institute; 2004.

Did You Know...

potassium, total protein, and calcium levels are lower in skin puncture blood than in venous blood.

8. Blood Culture

Alcohol prep before iodine for blood culture

I teach the phlebotomy class at my local hospital and am currently re-writing my lecture. The CLSI standard says to allow the site to air dry after cleansing with the disinfectant, then remove it from the skin with alcohol. Why should we clean the site with the alcohol after we have already sterilized it with chlorhexidine/povidone-iodine?

Also, do you have to clean the site initially with alcohol? Does it have to be a 2-part scrub at all? In the past we have used either chlorhexidine or povidone-iodine but not both. The kits we use come with a povidone-iodine swab for cleaning the arm. The alcohol wipe is used to clean the top of the collection bottles. Is this a "violation" if we only do a single scrub?

You are referring to an older version of the venipuncture standard. The newest version (H3-A6) doesn't include that reference. Instead, it states to remove iodine compounds from the skin after the procedure is complete to prevent absorption into the bloodstream and allergic reactions. It no longer mentions that it should be removed prior to the procedure. Historically, blood culture site prep has included an alcohol prep/scrub followed by a disinfectant such as iodine or chlorhexidine compounds. Recently a study showed three consecutive scrubs with 70% isopropyl alcohol to be just as effective as iodine in tincture form, povidone iodine, or povidone in combination with 70% ethyl alcohol.[1]

Regardless, the preliminary alcohol wipe is not as critical as a good friction scrub (30–60 seconds) to get to the bacteria beneath the dead skin cells on the surface. Nor is it as critical as assuring the antiseptic compound remains in contact with the skin for at least 30 seconds.

If you are using iodine or chlorhexidine compounds, it won't compromise the collection if the preliminary alcohol prep is left out. Again, the most critical aspect is friction and adequate skin contact with the disinfectant.

(cont...)

(Alcohol prep before iodine for blood culture cont...)

I wouldn't worry about "violating" the CLSI passage. But if you find your blood culture contamination rates creeping above 3% of all cultures collected, you might have to look at the lack of an alcohol prep step as one of the factors.

Reference

1) Calfee DP, Farr BM. Comparison of four antiseptic preparations for skin in the prevention of contamination of percutaneously drawn blood cultures: a randomized trial. *J Clin Microbiol* 2002 May;40(5):1660–5.

Did You Know...

if the alcohol used to cleanse the venipuncture
site is not dried before the puncture it will alter
results of the glucose, potassium, phosphorous
and uric acid as well as introduce a
hemolytic agent into the specimen.

Betadine substitute

We recently had a patient who had two sets of blood cultures ordered, but the patient had an allergy to betadine. Can you reference an article that details other acceptable forms for cleansing the site other than alcohol?

Your answer is to use a chlorhexidine compound or multiple scrubs with 70% isopropyl alcohol. As for references, the *Manual of Clinical Microbiology* talks about chlorhexidine as being superior as an antimicrobial and for having a low incidence of hypersensitivity. Other studies show chlorhexidine to be superior to povidone for blood culture prep.[1]

Researchers at the University of Virginia reported that three consecutive scrubs with 70% isopropyl alcohol were just as effective in preventing blood culture contamination as iodine in tincture form, povidone iodine, and povidone in combination with 70% ethyl alcohol.[2]

References

1) Mimoz O, Karim A, Mercat A, Cosseron M, et al. Chlorhexidine compared with povidone-iodine skin preparation before blood culture: a randomized controlled trial. *Annals Int Med* 1999;13(11):834–7.

2) Calfee DP, Farr BM. Comparison of four antiseptic preparations for skin in the prevention of contamination of percutaneously drawn blood cultures: a randomized trial. *J Clin Microbiol* 2002 May;40(5):1660–5.

Blood culture, cleansing stoppers

We have always cleansed our blood culture stoppers with iodine, and then removed the iodine with alcohol before filling them. A new employee is challenging us on that practice. What's the conventional wisdom on this?

The CLSI standards and most blood culture bottle manufacturers recommend an alcohol wipe only. You should check and follow what the manufacturer of your bottles recommends.

Blood cultures: drawing multiple sets

W hat's most important for blood culture collection: drawing each culture from a different site or assuring the proper volume is drawn?

A ccording to most blood culture authorities, it's considered more important to draw full volume blood cultures than to be concerned with spacing the draws apart. For adults, this means 20 cc per set divided between two bottles. Shorting the set can compromise the expediency of detecting and identifying organisms, which delays antibiotic therapy.

Allowing time to pass doesn't appear to be particularly necessary. Delaying the second set can affect the ability to harvest the causative organism of bacteremia. If the order was based on a fever spike, the population of the organism in the bloodstream peaked about 30 minutes before the fever spike. Any delay in collection decreases the chance of rapid bacterial detection and administration of antibiotics. So when blood cultures are ordered because of a fever spike, make sure they are collected as soon as possible. The bacteria are already on the decline *in vivo*.

Blood cultures from line draws

Q I'm having an argument with some of our staffers on blood cultures. They prefer to draw from a central line or arterial line if they can rather than to subject the patient to another stick. I disagree. What do you think? If I'm wrong, what is the best way to draw blood cultures from a central line?

A You're not wrong. There is no shortage of articles in the literature that advise against drawing cultures from vascular-access devices (VADs). VADs are notorious for contamination from bacteria that colonize around the cannula. Whenever drawing a set of blood cultures from a VAD, there must always be a set drawn by venipuncture to confirm/rule out the positive culture.

But here's the problem: if it so happens that the peripheral draw site was not adequately prepared or was contaminated by repalpation, then your patient has two false positive blood cultures, neither of which is from bacteria infecting the bloodstream. As a result, the physician is likely to give the patient antibiotics unnecessarily. Having said that, in many cases there are no options to drawing from VADs. In such cases, sterile technique plus a 5–10 cc discard will minimize the potential of a positive culture due to colonization, but it will never eliminate it completely.

Blood cultures from VADs:
prep & discard volume

How should a vascular-access device (VAD) be prepped before drawing a blood culture, and should blood there be a discard volume drawn before collecting the blood to be cultured? Our policy for the collection of blood cultures from vascular-access devices states "when collecting blood for culture, withdraw the amount of blood needed without wasting/discarding or flushing."

It's a good practice to discard the first 5 cc of blood from vascular-access devices to prevent contamination and interference from whatever is being infused. It would be good to challenge the procedure manual on this one as I believe one would be hard-pressed to find anything in the literature that says not to waste or discard prior to a blood draw.

As for prepping the device, the same technique should be used as if you were performing a venipuncture, i.e., at least 30 seconds of contact with the antiseptic before puncturing the device. You can forego the one-minute friction scrub since it's only applicable to skin.

Blood cultures in heparin tubes

When I am on the floor with a needle in a patient's arm and I'm paged to add a blood culture to the order, is it safe to use the green top for blood cultures? I know it is better to collect in the proper bottles, but there is a raging debate on this issue.

On the same subject, if we are sticking a baby with a fever for a CBC, we always draw a heparin tube for potential blood cultures to keep from resticking the child. Isn't this foresight in the best interest of the patient?

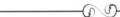

Actually, we're hard pressed to agree that such foresight is in the best interest of the patient. I know you are well meaning by not wanting to restick the patient, but in this case, you are doing the patient a disservice by straying from the standard for specimen collection. It's important to your patients to discontinue the practice for many reasons:

1.) Heparin is not a suitable anticoagulant for blood cultures.

2.) The stoppers of heparin tubes are not sterile.

3.) If the needle is already in the arm when you become aware of the order for blood cultures, more than likely the site was not properly prepped for a blood culture collection.

You have to be careful in phlebotomy not to reinvent the procedure by interjecting your own twists for the sake of expediency. Remember, your patient is depending on you to perform the procedure properly so that accurate results can be obtained from the specimens you draw. When you stray from the established procedure, you compromise the care the patient receives.

Blood cultures:
procedure for drawing two sets

I have two questions in regards to blood culture draws. The first includes the order in which you fill the aerobic vs. anaerobic bottles. Currently our hospital procedure is to draw the anaerobic bottle first so that air will not enter. However, the *Applied Phlebotomy Video Series* recommends filling the aerobic bottle first. Hopefully you can clarify for us the preferred order of blood cultures and what CLSI recommends.

The video is correct. The order depends on the equipment you use to draw the blood. If you are drawing into a syringe and then transferring the blood, you fill the anaerobic bottles first. This will prevent the inevitable air bubble that rises to the plunger interface from entering the anaerobic bottle. But if you are drawing through a butterfly directly into the bottles, as the video shows, you fill the aerobic vial first. If not, the air in the line will compromise the anaerobic environment.

A second reason for filling the aerobic vial first when drawing through a butterfly is to prevent a second puncture should the flow of blood stop and cannot be recovered prior to filling the second vial. An aerobic bottle will catch 98 percent of all bacteria that cause septicemia, whereas if you are only able to fill the anaerobic bottle, you'll need to restick the patient.

Blood culture reflux

Is there any danger when drawing blood culture bottles that the contents can reflux back into the patient? I had heard about this in a course a few years back, but have not found anything in literature. We are concerned about nurses using tube holders on central lines to draw blood cultures.

Reflux is always a concern. That's why the manufacturers of all but one blood culture system do not recommend filling bottles directly from a tube holder/needle assembly. Instead, the recommendation is to draw the blood through a butterfly attached to a tube holder or syringe, or directly into a syringe. Take a hard look at the manufacturer's instructions on the system you are using. If it doesn't specifically instruct you to draw directly into the bottle by placing it into the needle holder assembly as you would other blood collection tubes, don't.

Multiple blood cultures from one venipuncture

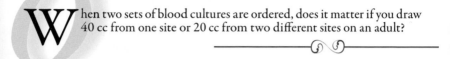

When two sets of blood cultures are ordered, does it matter if you draw 40 cc from one site or 20 cc from two different sites on an adult?

By definition, one blood culture is that blood which is drawn from one venipuncture. According to the American Society of Microbiology, when multiple bottles are filled from a single venipuncture, it constitutes a single blood culture.[1] The definition repeats in a revision of the same document published in 1997 along with a statement supporting the single-puncture/single-culture concept.[2] Finally, an article in the May, 1994 issue of *Laboratory Medicine* stated how increasingly apparent it is becoming that multiple venipunctures are as important for the diagnosis and treatment of bacteremia and fungemia in infants and older children as they are in adults.[3]

So a separate stick is clearly necessary and required. By inoculating two sets of bottles with blood from the same venipuncture, the interpretation of positive results becomes difficult. If there is growth in both sets, how do you know if the bacteria came from a skin contaminant or from the bloodstream? If your facility has a contamination rate of 2.2%, how do you classify alpha streps and coagulase-negative staphylococci that grow in all four bottles drawn from the same stick? Both organisms can be skin contaminants, but both can also be pathogenic. With just one stick, you eliminate an indicator that would help you interpret whether they are true or false positives.

(cont...)

(Multiple blood cultures from one venipuncture cont...)

References

1) Washington J, ed. *Blood Cultures II. Cumulative Techniques and Procedures in Clinical Microbiology.* ASM, 1982.

2) Hindler J, ed. *Blood Cultures III. Cumulative Techniques and Procedures in Clinical Microbiology.* ASM, 1997.

3) Kellogg, J, Ferrintino F, Liss J, Shapiro S, Bankert D. Justification and implementation of a policy requiring two blood cultures when one is ordered. *Lab Med* 1994;25(5):323–9.

Did You Know...

bacteremia involving E. coli can exist in the bloodstream in concentrations as low as one organism per ml of blood.

Site prep solutions for newborn blood cultures

The manufacturer of a chlorhexidine scrub says you cannot use the product on infants less than two months of age. Some of the nurses will not allow my phlebotomists to use betadine because they say this can harm the infant's skin. Our micro supervisor has heard that some places just prep with alcohol twice instead of using betadine. My infection control supervisor wants us to all come to a consensus on how to prep for infants. I cannot find any information on the Internet about betadine being harmful to infants. Can you share with me any information you have on this topic?

It's not so much that betadine is hard on neonatal skin as it is the risk iodine compounds pose to the thyroid and liver when it absorbs. Some facilities mitigate the risk by wiping the iodine off with isopropyl alcohol after the procedure.

Alternatively, you can use isopropyl alcohol alone as a prep solution. A study came out in 2002 that compared contamination rates of sites prepped with isopropyl alcohol three times, betadine, tincture iodine, and chlorhexidine and found them equivalent.[1]

However, isopropyl alcohol is considered to be harsh on neonatal skin.[2] Just remember, the key to a good prep is a 30-second friction scrub to get the antiseptic to come in contact with bacteria that could be under several layers of dead skin cells.

References

1) Calfee DP, Farr BM. Comparison of four antiseptic preparations for skin in the prevention of contamination of percutaneously drawn blood cultures: a randomized trial. *J Clin Microbiol* 2002 May;40(5):1660–5.

2) Lund C, Osborne J, Kuller J, Lane A, Lott J, Raines D. Neonatal skin care: clinical outcomes of the AWHONN/NANN evidence-based clinical practice guideline. *JOGNN* 2001;30(1):41–51.

Transporting blood cultures in a syringe

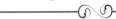

I see phlebotomists and other blood collection personnel collect blood cultures in a syringe, and then carry it all the way to the (microbiology) lab where they then dispense it into the appropriate blood culture media. This could be because they did not have the media at the point of collection. Is this acceptable considering the sterility issue, the potential for micro-clots to form, and the safety compromised during specimen transportation?

This practice is not likely to compromise results if the only test being performed on the blood in the syringe is the blood culture. Bacteria will grow whether the blood is clotted or not. However, it may be a safety issue for two reasons. First, if the collector is carrying the device with the needle exposed, the risk is obvious. (Even if they activate the safety feature on the needle immediately upon collection, it's still not optimum.)

The second risk is that, by the time the collector arrives to the micro department, the blood is clotted in the barrel or the hub of the syringe. If so, the collector might be tempted to push on the plunger to force the blood into the culture bottle. The risk is that the safety transfer device (assuming they've replaced the needle with the device as is required) can explode off of the syringe, and blood could splatter the face and garments.

The facility that nurtures a culture of safety does not allow blood to be transported in a syringe (unless it is a blood gas, of course), and insists all blood be evacuated into the appropriate tubes or bottles at the patient's side.

Tube holders for large blood culture bottles

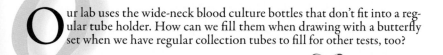

ur lab uses the wide-neck blood culture bottles that don't fit into a regular tube holder. How can we fill them when drawing with a butterfly set when we have regular collection tubes to fill for other tests, too?

arger size tube holders are available for wide-neck bottles. Contact the bottle manufacturer and ask for them. They come with an insert so that, after you fill the blood culture bottle, you insert a sleeve into the tube holder to accommodate tubes for other lab work. They have the wide-neck safety transfer devices for syringe draws, too.

9. Labeling & Post-Venipuncture Care

Labeling
Acceptable number of mislabeled specimens
Disciplining personnel who mislabel specimens
Prelabeling tubes
Specimen labeling by hand

Post-Venipuncture Care
Arterial pressure
Bandaging
Bruising stats
Gauze wraps
Hematoma prevention
Obese patients and bending the elbow
Patients bending the arm up after a venipuncture
Preventing hematoma formation
Spot bandages on coumadin patients
Thumb versus finger for applying pressure

Acceptable number of mislabeled specimens

I have been a Medical Technologist for over 30 years. Misidentification was a problem when I first began and it continues to be one today. One of our facilities is being told that limiting a phlebotomist to two validated patient identification errors of major consequence is too stringent. They allow up to five errors of minor consequence.

I find this very frustrating. Are there are any standards that address the number of mislabeled samples that can be considered acceptable? Do you have any specific regulatory references that would assist this facility?

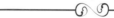

The acceptable number of mislabeled specimens is zero. The facility would be hard-pressed to find one reputable supervisor, authority, text, article or regulation that states it acceptable to have even one mislabeled specimen. It is imperative that you hold to your high standards and apply them facility-wide. You may well be some patient's last line of defense. Every patient, present and future, is counting on you to stand firm so that they may be protected.

As to the number an employee is allowed before termination, that is up to the facility. No precedent exists in the literature, nor are there any limits established by any regulating agency to my knowledge. I would call upon your risk manager for reinforcement.

Disciplining personnel
who mislabel specimens

We have been experiencing many labeling errors by our phlebotomists, and have terminated several in the last few months. Do you have any suggestions as to how we can resolve these issues? The phlebotomy technicians that we have had to let go were very hard-working, experienced people. We do yearly competencies; I personally train people and I just can't understand this. Please give me some suggestions.

I know you don't like terminating otherwise good employees, but you are doing the right thing if they continue to disregard proper labeling policies. One way to get your staff to understand the importance is by giving them reminders in as many forms as possible. Use your bulletin boards, mention it at every inservice, put fliers that remind them in their paychecks or department mail boxes, send them emails periodically. It doesn't have to be punitive in tone, but make the messages fun while being serious about the point. Use clip art cartoon figures, create a mascot (for example: "Just a reminder from 'the Identi-Fly', are you labeling all specimens at the patient's side?") ... things like that.

CLSI now requires that collectors perform a final check of the arm bracelet against the labels on the tubes before leaving the patient. Alternatively the patient can be asked to verify that the tubes are labeled correctly.

Prelabeling tubes

I s it acceptable to prelabel all collection tubes with the patient's information, prior to performing a venipuncture?

N ot at all. The standards are solidly against this practice. The risk is that labeled but unused tubes could be inadvertently left behind and accidentally used on another patient.

Let's say it's your practice to prelabel tubes before the draw. The venipuncture is unsuccessful after two attempts and you leave the inpatient's room, forgetting to discard the tubes from your tray. (Or, worse yet, leaving them in the room for someone else to use.) You've created a situation that opens the door for all kinds of medical mistakes.

If you look at the CLSI venipuncture standard (H3), it lists in chronological order the steps of the venipuncture procedure. Labeling tubes is step 15, which comes after the specimen is drawn. Later in the document, it states that the labels should be placed on the tubes after collection is complete. Finally, it states the tubes must not be labeled before they are filled. So it's quite clear that prelabeling is not acceptable. You should work to establish firm language in your policies against prelabeling.

Specimen labeling by hand

Is it acceptable to label a tube by hand, then apply a permanent label later when you have more time?

Handwriting on the tube label is fine as long as it is done after the tubes are filled and includes all the proper information. And of course all specimens must be labeled at the patient's side. No exceptions. None. According to CLSI document H3, the completed label must be attached to the tube after the draw and before leaving the side of the patient. Later in the document it states that the collector must compare the labeled tube to the identification bracelet, or have the patient confirm that it was properly labeled whenever possible.

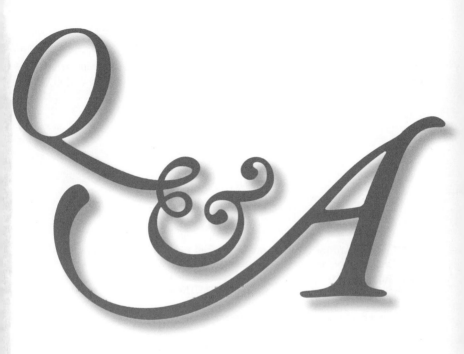

Arterial pressure

Q Is there a recommended time standard for applying pressure to the artery during either a routine stick for blood gases or an inadvertent arterial puncture? Does the standard apply to laboratories only or does it apply to physician office draws, too?

A The standard for pressure on an arterial puncture is 3–5 minutes, then check for bleeding and hematoma formation and apply additional pressure if necessary.[1] The standard is the same regardless of who draws the specimen or the type of facility they work in. The standards are established by the Clinical and Laboratory Standards Institute (CLSI) (www.clsi.org) and should be reflected in any procedure manual.

Reference

1) CLSI. *Procedures for the Collection of Arterial Blood Specimens; Approved Standard— Fourth Edition*. CLSI document H11-A4. Wayne, PA: Clinical and Laboratory Standards Institute; 2004.

Bandaging

Whaat is your opinion regarding taping the patient's arm? (i.e., using the gauze and taping it to the arm). I have staff who thinks taping gauze to the site shouldn't be done for in-patients because of the frequency of phlebotomy on these patients. They argue that the tape damages the skin when removed.

Bandaging should be done, whether using tape, an adhesive bandage, or a commercial wrap that secures the gauze in place without an adhesive. Wounds should not be left uncovered. If your staff is concerned about the effect of tape on patients, you might want to try hypoallergenic tape or a gauze wrap such as Coban™ or Kerlix™ for those frequently drawn patients.

Coban™ is a trademark of 3M™.
Kerlix™ is a trademark of Covidien-Kendall.

Bruising stats

Do you have a source for what the average bruise rate should be when performing phlebotomy? ────────────

AQ-Probe published in 1991 examined patient satisfaction and complications among 30,000 patients (80% survey return rate).[1] The survey gathered data on the size (average: 15.1 mm) and frequency (16.1%) of bruising and the number of attempts by phlebotomists per patient (1.03). Ninety-three percent of venipunctures were eventually successful (4.9% not attempted). But it doesn't state how many attempts were made before they were successful.

A CAP Q-Probe conducted in 1992 addressed the level of recollects at 70 hospitals: 95% were collected on first attempt; 2.8% required two attempts; 0.8% required three attempts and 1.1% required four or more sticks.[2] Unfortunately, this data is a bit dated. We haven't seen any more recent studies published.

References

1) Howantiz P, Cembrowski G, Bachner P. Laboratory phlebotomy. *Arch Pathol Lab Med* 1991;115:867–872.

2) Howantiz P, Schifman R. Inpatient phlebotomy practices: A College of American Pathologists Q-Probe study of 2,351,643 phlebotomy requests. *Arch Pathol Lab Med* 1994;118:601–605.

Gauze wraps

Our outpatient phlebotomists have begun to use an adhesive gauze wrap as a pressure bandage on our routine outpatients. It seems that our patients are asking for it, thinking that it is better than regular tape, but the question came up that there could be liability if the patient does not remove it in a timely manner. Do you have any information and/or references regarding the use of this type of product?

Unless the stretchy gauze wrap is applied so tightly that it restricts circulation, there shouldn't be any problems associated with a prolonged application. Maybe an in-service would be in order to demonstrate how loosely it should be applied as a way to manage the risk. Another way to limit your liability is to give the patient written post-venipuncture care instructions that tell when to remove the wrap. You might contact the manufacturer for proper use instructions.

Hematoma prevention

I am looking for any study showing the use of cohesive bandages like Coban™ on patients on heparin or coumadin. Have you ever seen a study or recommendation to support their use?

No, but their use makes good sense. Just make sure you and those who work with you and for you don't consider such wraps as a substitute for applying pressure or observing the site prior to application.

Use it in conjunction with the practice of observing the site for hematoma formation for several seconds (5–10) after releasing pressure, but before applying the wrap. Too many folks are in such a hurry to bandage that they don't take time to observe for bleeding beneath the surface of the skin. To them, a wrap might be considered as a substitute for that step, and allow collectors to think that any bleeding will be well absorbed by the wrap.

There should be a two-point check for bleeding: look for bleeding from the puncture site and also for hematoma formation. Failing to observe for hematoma formation beneath the surface of the skin can cause serious complications, including nerve injury. In the CLSI venipuncture standard, this observation step is required for all patients, not just those on blood thinner.

Coban™ is a trademark of 3M™.

Obese patients and bending the elbow

Do you have specific tips for locating veins in obese patients? One of our employees sticks obese patients with the patient's elbow bent. I can see bending it slightly while palpating for a vein, but I wouldn't stick a patient with their elbow bent. Would you?

Relaxing the joint slightly is acceptable, but only slightly. Bending the elbow can be taught as a possible means of locating vein that can't be found when the elbow is locked, but the technique is not unique to obese patients. Even normal-weight patients can have veins that only appear visibly or palpably when the elbow is slightly bent. It's not necessary for the elbow to be completely locked so that the arm is rigidly straight.

Patients bending the arm up after a venipuncture

Most of our phlebotomists have the patient bend the arm up to facilitate clotting. I recently had a nurse comment that she heard it was not appropriate. Who's right?

The nurse is correct. Bending the arm up is not an adequate substitute for pressure and can lead to a hematoma. Besides being unsightly, hematomas can lead to nerve damage by placing pressure on the nerves. According to the CLSI standards, direct pressure is required.

The patient may be recruited to apply pressure, but it is ultimately the collector's responsibility to assure pressure is adequate. To assure adequate pressure, the collector can observe the nail beds of the patient's fingers that are applying pressure. If they are whitish, it's a strong indication that he/she is pressing down hard enough. If the nail beds of the finger(s) applying pressure remain pinkish, pressure is probably inadequate. The collector must, therefore, be prepared to take over if the patient doesn't seem to be applying enough pressure.

Preventing hematoma formation

I drew blood from an elderly woman using a 22g needle and a tube holder. I needed two gold tops and one purple top. The first gold top filled fine, but when I switched tubes, a hematoma was forming and I had to take the needle out.

Why do hematomas form during a blood draw? Would it have helped to use a butterfly instead of a 22-gauge needle? Is it possible that during the switching of tubes in the holder that I moved the needle out of position causing the hematoma? What can I do to prevent this from happening in the future?

The hematoma was likely a result of two things: the age of the patient and needle movement during tube exchange. Elderly patients are more prone to hematoma formation than younger patients. That's because when you puncture a vein of a younger patient, the vein is more elastic and constricts around the needle when it is inserted. In older patients, the elasticity is gone and the blood readily oozes from the vein where the needle passes though its upper wall. Should the needle be disrupted during tube exchange, as is likely in your case, the space around the needle increases and the hematoma forms.

You can minimize the oozing of blood around the needle by keeping the needle as stationary as possible during the transfer. Keep the backs of your fingers holding the syringe or tube holder firmly on the patient's forearm, and make sure you use the flared extensions of the device to push on and pull off the tubes.

Spot bandages on coumadin patients

Recently I have noticed the phlebotomists at my facility using spot bandages on coumadin patients. Before I let my manager know about it, I want to make sure I'm not missing something. Are pressure bandages not in vogue any more? Do CLSI standards address this issue? Are there other sources I should refer to?

CLSI doesn't say anything about pressure bandages, even for coumadin patients. It only says the collector must bandage the patient after observing for hematoma formation, being sure stasis is complete. You are right to be concerned, though. One little bump to the arm of an overmedicated coumadin patient could dislodge the fragile fibrin plug sealing the venipuncture site and lead to profuse bleeding.

If your manager is proactive, you might suggest a change in policy for coumadin patients. If not, you might have to wait for a victim to return to the lab with a bloody arm. You are to be commended for keeping the best interests of the patient in mind.

Thumb versus finger for applying pressure

What is the difference between using the thumb versus the index finger to hold the gauze in place when withdrawing the needle? I like the students to use the index finger because:

1.) They are less likely to press too hard before the needle has actually exited the arm; (students seem to have more control of the index finger versus the thumb).

2.) The pressure would start to be applied ahead (away from) the actual needle exit point with the index finger, rather than over the exit point with the thumb;

3.) They are less likely to poke themselves, as the thumb is actually closer to the exiting needle than the index finger would be;

4.) I like the looks of it.

This could be argued either way. The index finger seems more like the natural way to apply pressure. Using the thumb sounds awkward. Since nothing is written on it, it's personal preference. Your rationale makes perfect sense.

10. Line Draws & IV Starts

Discouraging draws during IV starts
Drawing from a line infused with TPA
Drawing from triple lumen catheters
Draws from saline locks
Draws from VADs
Hemoglobin variations in line draws
Hooking an IV up to a butterfly set
How do I limit draws during IV starts in the ED?
Nurses and line draws
Phlebotomists doing line draws
Phlebotomists starting IVs
Vascular access draws

Discouraging draws during IV starts

I am wondering if you have any articles, studies, or opinions on the practice of collecting blood during IV starts? I am preparing to provide in-depth phlebotomy training to a group of nursing assistants, but anticipate that they may resort to IV-start collections instead.

───────────────── ❦ ❦ ─────────────────

Vascular access devices (VADs) are notorious for hemolyzing blood specimens. The biggest problem occurs in emergency rooms where the staff routinely withdraws specimens during an IV start. Hemolysis is inherent with such devices.

Try to discourage this as best you can. You might run up against the argument that it saves time, but counter with the time lost when specimens have to be recollected due to hemolysis. Explain that when you draw blood through a VAD, you are using the device for a purpose for which it was not designed. They are made for fluids to be infused into the patient, not for blood to be withdrawn. The shear forces and turbulence at the tip of the cannula are too extreme for the fragile red blood cells to tolerate. Hemolysis affects every analyte that could be tested because when a specimen is hemolyzed, what was once solid (RBCs) is now liquid. So there's a dilutional affect to all analytes, not to mention the interference of free hemoglobin and cellular materials.

There's not much that can be done to minimize hemolysis during IV starts other than to avoid such draws altogether. However, there are plenty of articles and studies in the existing literature that you might find helpful. Here's a summary:

- A study found a significant increase in the hemolysis rate in blood drawn during IV starts than by venipuncture, 13.7% versus 3.8% respectively.[1]

- A study showing hemolysis in ED samples drawn by venipuncture was <1%, while those drawn during IV starts was 20%.[2]

(cont...)

(Discouraging draws during IV starts cont...)

- The same study compared hemolysis rates when specimens were drawn through IV catheters using a syringe (9%) versus a tube holder/vacuum tube combination (22%).[2] Another study showed the difference to be 3 versus 19% respectively.[3]

- A study showed the difference in hemolysis rates between specimens drawn from ED personnel versus laboratory phlebotomists to be 12.4% (ED personnel) versus 1.6% (phlebotomists).[4]

- A study showing hemolysis of samples drawn during IV starts using 5 ml tubes was nearly 50% lower than when samples were collected in the same manner using 10 ml tubes (1.1% versus 2% respectively).[5]

- A study showed blood drawn through 20–24 gauge IV catheters was more than seven times as likely to be hemolyzed than that drawn through 14–16 gauge cannulas, and 3.6 times as likely as blood drawn through an 18-gauge cannula.[6]

References

1) Kennedy C, Angermuller S, King R, Noviello S, Walker J, et al. A comparison of hemolysis rates using intravenous catheters versus venipuncture tubes for obtaining blood samples. *J Emerg Nurs* 1996 22(6):566–569.

2) Grant M. The effect of blood drawing techniques and equipment on the hemolysis of ED laboratory blood samples. *J Emerg Nurs* 2003;29(2):116–21.

3) Stankovic A, Smith S. Elevated serum potassium values: the role of Preanalytic variables. *Am J Clin Pathol* 2004;121(Suppl1):S105–Sl12 5105.

4) Burns E, Yoshikawa N. Hemolysis in serum samples drawn by emergency department personnel versus laboratory phlebotomists. *Lab Med* 2002;5(33):378–80.

5) Cox S, Dages J, Jarjoura D, Hazelett S. Blood samples drawn from IV catheters have less hemolysis when 5-ml (vs 10-ml) collection tubes are used. *J Emerg Nurs* 2004;30(6):529–33.

6) Tenabe P. Letter to the editor. *J Emerg Nurs* 2004;30(2):106–8.

Drawing from a line infused with TPA

When TPA is being given into a triple-lumen catheter, we flush with 20 mL of saline, and discard 10 mL of blood. We are finding that we have unreliable results. Should we collect from one of the opposite cannulas or refuse to collect from the device period? If we opt to draw from the line, what is the appropriate protocol?

Neither textbooks nor the CLSI standard address the administration of the clot-buster medications like TPA (tissue plasminogen activator) in the context of a line draw. But it makes sense to have a policy that states all ports of a line into which TPA is administered should be off limits. As evidenced by your own experience with skewed results, even flushing and discarding large volumes doesn't guarantee a clean specimen.

Drawing from the opposite arm would be preferable. If not possible, draw below the IV on the same arm. Regardless of where you perform the venipuncture, pressure to the site should be applied and bleeding carefully guarded prior to bandaging.

Drawing from triple lumen catheters

With a triple lumen catheter, there is one port that is used to draw blood. Do all other ports need to be shut off for a certain amount of time before collecting the specimen, and should there be a volume discarded before withdrawing blood to be tested?

According to the Infusion Nurses Society's *Procedures and Policies for Infusion Nursing*, the procedure for withdrawing blood from a triple lumen catheter is the same as what the CLSI venipuncture standard says for drawing from any vascular-access device. That is, all other ports need to be shut off for at least two minutes. The lumen through which the blood is to be drawn should be flushed with 5 cc of saline, and a discard volume withdrawn prior to collecting the specimen. The discard volume should be twice the dead-space volume of the catheter for all labs except coags, which require six times the dead-space volume. 5 cc is usually sufficient.

You should confirm this with your facility's policy and make sure the policy squares with the standards.

Draws from saline locks

I would like to know if most labs draw blood from saline locks, especially during post-thrombolytic therapy.

Saline or heparin locks are tricky to draw from. An article published in the September 1999 issue of *American Journal of Critical Care* concludes that 18-gauge saline locks are suitable for drawing coagulation studies with a 0.5 cc discard.[1] No significant difference in the aPTT or PT levels was observed between the blood drawn from the saline lock and blood drawn by venipuncture at the same time. The authors state that collectors did not experience any problems with any of the draws.

Reference

1) Arrants J, Willis M, Stevens B, Gripkey L, et al. Reliability of an intravenous intermittent access port (saline lock) for obtaining blood samples for coagulation studies. *Am J Crit Care* 1999;8(5):344–348.

Draws from VADs

W hat is the common practice for drawing coagulation specimens from venous-access devices? I know CLSI has issued guidelines for this procedure that recommend flushing with 5 mL of saline and discarding the first 5 mL of blood or six times the dead space of the catheter. Is it appropriate to follow these standards routinely, or only when no other venipuncture site can be found? Phlebotomists are put in a challenging position when patients request their line be used, but nurses insist specimens be drawn by venipuncture.

T he standards promoted by the Clinical and Laboratory Standards Institute (CLSI) discuss how to draw from a vascular-access device (VAD), not when. It's best to avoid VAD draws because of the increased potential for preanalytical error from contamination, hemolysis, etc., and to draw from them only when no veins are accessible. When doctors tell patients that their VAD will prevent them from having to endure venipunctures, it becomes a problem for those with blood collection responsibilities who know the risk line draws pose to accurate results. There's no easy answer for this dilemma except to explain to the physician the problem that such a comment to the patient presents.

Hemoglobin variations in line draws

I am the phlebotomy coordinator in a large hospital in Australia. We are having a problem with erroneous results from our oncology department where blood is collected from central venous catheters by the nursing staff. On one patient, the haemoglobin rose from 117 g/L to 171 g/L in 24 hours, then came back down two hours later to 109 g/L. There was no transfusion and tourniquet application was not prolonged. This happens a lot. The nursing staff discards 10 mL before collecting samples. Can you explain such a difference?

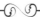

In order to address this variation fairly, we have to question the accuracy of both the normal and abnormal results. In other words, we have to wonder if the normal result is falsely lower or if the higher result is falsely elevated. There are more explanations for a falsely lower hemoglobin drawn from a line than a falsely elevated result. Variables that falsely decrease hemoglobins from line draws include dilution with IV fluids, clotting in the barrel of the syringe prior to filling the tubes, and hemolysis during aspiration. You should investigate if the nurses are turning off the fluids for two minutes prior to collection. If not, there could be a dilutional effect.

Variables that falsely elevate hemoglobin in line draws include hemoconcentration, which most commonly occurs when the tourniquet is left on for a prolonged time. You've ruled that out. Physiological conditions like dehydration can also falsely elevate hemoglobin. But if the level came back down two hours later, dehydration is probably not the issue unless it was rapidly corrected by IV infusion between sampling.

Make sure your specimens are well mixed prior to testing. Check the EDTA tubes for clots. Observation of the nurses' technique may reveal other variables. Finally, make sure this is not an analytical (instrumentation) issue instead of a preanalytical issue. You might want to confirm all spurious results by repeat testing.

Hooking an IV up to a butterfly set

There is a nurse in our clinic who is having problems starting IVs. She would like to have our phlebotomist access the vein with a butterfly, and then she will connect her IV to the set. I have never heard of such a thing, and I don't think it is legal. Isn't this putting the phlebotomist in the position of starting an IV? If you can find any standards or documentation that I could show this nurse, I would appreciate it.

The butterfly sets your phlebotomist is carrying around are not likely designed for infusion therapy. The steel needles of a winged blood collection set are not intended to be left in place. Your phlebotomist should resist.

If the nurse is requesting the phlebotomist insert an IV set for infusing fluids, that's probably not a good idea either, unless the phlebotomist is trained on IV insertion.

Bring this issue to the attention of your nurse manager. She may not be aware of the intent to rig a blood collection device for IV infusion. At the same time, instruct your phlebotomists to resist such requests since merging these two procedures may not be advisable. As a phlebotomist, it's well within his/her right to resist any attempt by someone from another department to modify the blood collection procedure. Resistance should continue until and unless research proves it's a recognized modification in the industry and one that is supported in the facility's procedure manual. If the facility permits it, it should be reflected in both laboratory and nursing procedure manuals. You might also have your nurse manager check the modification against nursing policies and the standards of the Infusion Nurses Society.

If you need more ammunition, you can always contact the manufacturer of the device the nurse is trying to use for double duty. If the manufacturer frowns on it, you must, too. It's about liability. You don't want a jury to have to consider the consequences for using a device against manufacturer's recommendations. Your risk manager will likely be an ally to your cause.

How do I limit draws during IV starts in the ED?

How can I convince our emergency department (ED) not to draw blood during an IV start? We have a high rate of hemolysis in ED specimens and I have tracked it down to specimens drawn through an IV while it is being inserted, before the fluids are started.

Preventing hemolysis in the ED is probably the most common specimen collection problem hospitals face. This much is indisputable: if you have an emergency room, you have a hemolysis problem! The only facilities that don't are those that perform venipunctures for all their ED lab work. You will always have a problem with hemolysis as long as blood is drawn during IV starts. Sometimes you can get away with it; sometimes you can't. The problem is that when blood is drawn through a VAD, the device is being used for a purpose for which it was not intended. The shear forces and turbulence surrounding the tip of the cannula are too much for the fragile red cells.

The literature is packed with studies that prove hemolysis is difficult to avoid during a line draw. Some of them are listed below. Inform your ED that hemolysis is an inherent problem with draws during IV starts. Explain that, although their intent to save the patient a stick is well-intended, too many times the patient has to endure a forced delay in testing and reporting due to recollections. Let them know studies have shown significant increases in hemolysis in samples obtained through IV catheters versus venipunctures. As long as they insist on drawing blood during an IV start they will have hemolyzed specimens.

Bibliography

- Kennedy C, Angermuller S, King R, Noviello S, Walker J, et al. A comparison of hemolysis rates using intravenous catheters versus venipuncture tubes for obtaining blood samples. *J Emerg Nurs* 1996 22(6):566–569.

(cont...)

(How do I limit draws during IV starts in the ED? cont...)

- Herr R, Bossart P, Blaylock R, Kroger K, Owen J. Intravenous catheter aspiration for obtaining basis analysis during intravenous infusion. *Ann Emerg Med* 1990;19:789–92.

- Grant M. The effect of blood drawing techniques and equipment on the hemolysis of ED laboratory blood samples. *J Emerg Nurs* 2003;29(2):116–21.

- Stankovic A, Smith S. Elevated serum potassium values: the role of Preanalytic variables. *Am J Clin Pathol* 2004;121(Suppl1):S105–Sl12 5105.

- Burns E, Yoshikawa N. Hemolysis in serum samples drawn by emergency department personnel versus laboratory phlebotomists. *Lab Med* 2002;5(33):378–80.

- Cox S, Dages J, Jarjoura D, Hazelett S. Blood samples drawn from IV catheters have less hemolysis when 5 mL (vs 10 mL) collection tubes are used. *J Emerg Nurs* 2004;30(6):529–33.

- Tenabe P. Letter to the editor. *J Emerg Nurs* 2004;30(2):106–8.

- Lowe G, Stike R, Pollack M, Bosley J, O'Brien P, et al. Nursing blood specimen collection techniques and hemolysis rates in an emergency department: analysis of venipuncture versus intravenous catheter collection techniques. *J Emerg Nurs* 2008;34(1):26–32.

- Dugan L, Leech L, Speroni K, Corriher J. Factors affecting hemolysis rates in blood samples drawn from newly placed IV sites in the emergency department. *J Emerg Nurs* 2005;31(4):338–45.

- Ernst D. *Applied Phlebotomy.* Lippincott Williams & Wilkins. Philadelphia, PA. 2005.

Nurses and line draws

I'm looking for literature that will provide me with knowledge enough to train nurses on proper technique for getting blood specimens from PICC lines, central lines, arterial lines, etc. We are having problems with some point-of-care testing results not correlating with results from specimens drawn from lines. Any thoughts?

There's quite a lot of information out there on line draws, but it all is based on the standards as set forth by the Clinical and Laboratory Standards Institute (CLSI). The Infusion Nurses Society policies and procedures reflect these standards as well. According to CLSI, you should avoid drawing through lines if at all possible. If not possible to avoid, the line should be flushed with 5 mL of saline, and the first 5 mL of blood or six dead-space volumes of the vascular-access device (VAD) discarded if you're drawing coagulation tests. Discarding two times the dead-space volume is recommended for noncoagulation testing. For additional information, please refer to:

- CLSI. *Collection, Transport, and Processing of Blood Specimens for Testing Plasma-Based Coagulation Assays and Molecular Hemostasis Assays; Approved Guideline—Fifth Edition.* CLSI document H21-A5. Wayne, PA: Clinical and Laboratory Standards Institute; 2008.

- CLSI. *Procedures for the Collection of Diagnostic Blood Specimens by Venipuncture; Approved Standard—Sixth Edition.* CLSI document H3-A6. Wayne, PA: Clinical and Laboratory Standards Institute; 2007.

The standards serve as the basis for any laboratory procedure, including phlebotomy, and apply to all healthcare personnel. As you know, the standards are the standards regardless of what profession is performing the procedure and, according to the Clinical Laboratory Improvement Amendments passed in 1988 (CLIA '88), the laboratory is responsible for the quality of the specimens it tests.

CLSI document H3 is available as an immediate download or as a bound booklet from the Center for Phlebotomy Education's web site (www.phlebotomy.com). Bound copies of H3 and H21 can be purchased and shipped from CLSI directly (www.clsi.org).

Phlebotomists doing line draws

Q ur neurovascular intensive care nurses request phlebotomists learn to take blood from lines. What do you think of this idea? Have you ever heard of other hospitals actually doing this?

U nless you are in a state that regulates who can and can't manage infusions, it's not likely that there are any legal implications in training phlebotomists to do line draws. Generally, any employer can train any employee to perform the procedure as long as they provide adequate training. The onus is on the employer to develop a training regimen that protects the patient from complications. It's rare in the industry for phlebotomists to be trained to draw blood from lines without nursing supervision.

Phlebotomists starting IVs

We have always been told it is not in a phlebotomist's "scope of practice" to legally be able to start IVs or start any type of vascular-access devices or draw from/flush any of these devices. Is this really a law?

Phlebotomy is a very unregulated profession. As such, it does not have a widely accepted scope of practice as other professions do defining the procedures they can perform. Even if it did, a scope of practice would state what a professional in that field could do, not what he/she cannot.

Some states have legislation that requires specimen collection personnel to be certified (California, Nevada, and to a lesser extent, Louisiana), but if a hospital or healthcare facility wants to assign a phlebotomist to start IVs, there's not likely to be a law that restricts their ability to do so. However, should an injury result and the patient sue, the employer will have to prove the person starting the IV was properly trained and regularly evaluated. Without convincing evidence, it may not be possible to prove that the facility adequately protected the patient population from injury.

So if a facility is going to give its phlebotomists a procedure that is not typical for the profession, it must make sure training is adequate and the procedure is in the employee's job description to fully protect itself. Phlebotomists are often called upon to withdraw blood from vascular-access devices such as IV lines, central (IV) lines and arterial lines, but in most cases they assist the nursing staff in the procedure and are not performing the procedure themselves.

IV management is a highly complex procedure with significant risk to the patient if not undertaken with comprehensive training. So it's critical that facilities that want to expand the phlebotomist's role to include drawing specimens from vascular-access devices without supervision do so with a great deal of training, oversight, and regular evaluations. Just like there's a lot more to phlebotomy than accessing a vein, so too for IVs.

Vascular access draws

Our nurses are balking at discarding a calculated volume of blood when drawing specimens from a line. They say it's not in their standards that way and they want proof. They are saying the same thing for the order of draw, especially in regards to the citrate (blue top) tube. Can you help?

——————————— ✑ ✑ ———————————

Actually, it is in their standards. Have them refer to those ascribed by their own Infusion Nurses Society under "Blood Specimen Collection from Vascular-Access Devices."

Not that it matters, because anyone drawing specimens for clinical testing must conform to the standards in effect by the testing facility. The laboratory is responsible for the quality of the specimens it tests (a CLIA '88 statement). The standard is the same, regardless of the qualifications of the person drawing the specimen, and deviations from standards should be disciplined uniformly.

The pertinent CLSI standards are document H21, *Collection, Transport, and Processing of Blood Specimens for Coagulation Testing and General Performance of Coagulation Assays and Molecular Hemostasis Assays* and document H3, *Procedures for the Collection of Diagnostic Blood Specimens by Venipuncture.* The latter is available on the Center for Phlebotomy Education's web site as an immediate download. (www.phlebotomy.com/Downloads.html.) Each document states that about 5 mL of blood must be discarded whenever drawing through a vascular-access device.

As for the order of draw for citrate tubes, document H3 places the citrate tube before the serum tube. Should your nurses place it at the end of the order, they risk carrying over EDTA or (worse) heparin into the coag tube and erroneous results. By placing it at the end of the line, there is a significant potential that the aPTT and/or protime result will be erroneously lengthened and an undermedicated patient may appear well within therapeutic range. Do they want to be responsible for the patient throwing a clot or stroking out? That's the risk they are putting on the patient by not sticking to established standards for specimen collection. If a tactful, cooperative approach won't work, bring in the risk manager.

Finally, laboratory managers who knowingly permit results to be reported from improperly drawn specimens can bring substantial liability on the laboratory, even if a disclaimer accompanies the result.[1] Deviating from the standard is a huge liability. You are probably the patient's last line of defense against medical mistakes that could have catastrophic consequences. First be tactful; then be firm. Your patients are depending on you.

Reference

1) Harty-Golder B. Liability and the lab. *MLO* 2004;36(9):43.

Did You Know...
excessive crying can temporarily
elevate white blood cell counts in infants.

11. Processing, Storage, & Transportation

Processing

Acceptance of uncentrifuged specimens

Clotting time before centrifugation

Glucose stability on gel

How long can tubes sit before centrifugation?

Storage & Transportation

Affects of storage on EDTA specimens

Chilling serum tubes during transportation

Icing blood gas specimens

LDH and storage

Phosphorous and preanalytical errors

Regulation of specimen transport

Specimen stability in a cooler

Stability of CBC values and sed rates

Thawed specimens

Transporting aPTTs

Transporting protimes

Unspun chemistries & coags

Acceptance of uncentrifuged specimens

Do you have any comments on how long a clot tube should clot before being processed? I wait until I see retraction of the clot, but a phlebotomist from another state rejects the specimen if it isn't spun before transporting by courier. (It's a 15-mile trip to the lab.) In both cases, the labs are pretty small, and the specimen will not get caught in a queue of batched specimens. Any ideas would be appreciated.

Clot retraction might be a good indicator, but it may not always be reliable. Complete clotting can take up to 30 minutes. If centrifuged prematurely, the lab may have to deal with fibrin strands, which can cause problems with automated processing systems. Most manufacturers recommend spinning tubes 20–30 minutes after collection. For those specimens drawn moments before your courier arrives, centrifugation may be hurried and lead to hemolysis and forced recentrifugation.

As long as clotted specimens arrive at the facility and can be centrifuged within two hours of collection, they should be fine. Just make sure unspun specimens aren't transported at refrigerated temperatures. Refrigeration is for vegetables, not uncentrifuged chemistry specimens. If specimens are not centrifuged within two hours, or are transported at refrigerated temperatures before centrifugation, the potassiums will not likely be accurate. Red cells have 23 times more potassium than the serum or plasma does. What keeps the potassium in the cells is what's known as the sodium-ATPase pump. At refrigerated temperatures, the pump slows and potassium rushes out of the cells into the serum or plasma. Even if kept at room temperature during transportation, the values cannot be considered reliable if more than two hours have passed since collection. The tech should be applauded for rejecting uncentrifuged specimens for this reason.

It's my guess the tech on the receiving end assumes all uncentrifuged specimens are transported refrigerated. Specimen rejection would then be understandable and appropriate. Perhaps a conversation with the testing facility would be in order to see if their policy can accommodate the acceptance of just-drawn specimens provided they are kept at room temperature and received in the testing facility within two hours per CLSI recommendations.

Clotting time before centrifugation

What is the length of time for a red top or SST to sit before spinning once it looks clotted?

Complete clotting can take up to 30 minutes. Sometimes a specimen looks clotted because it doesn't flow in the tube when you invert it, but that may not be a good measure that complete clotting has taken place. The clot may still be forming within the partially congealed specimen. Don't fall victim to the myth that a clot activator accelerates clotting. Activators facilitate complete clotting, not faster clotting. Even though clot activator tubes may gel up quickly, complete clotting can still take up to 30 minutes.

If you find a lot of your specimens have fibrin in the serum after centrifugation, it's an indication you are rushing things. Set a clock for 20–30 minutes and see if the problem goes away. Of course patients on anticoagulants or with a coagulopathy may take longer.

Glucose stability on gel

A bout how long would glucose be stable in a gel barrier tube that was centrifuged and stored for six days? Some here are arguing the gel barrier protects the glucose; I think that the glucose leaches into the gel, causing a falsely low result. Can you provide me with the proper info and a reference?

A ccording to CLSI, serum stored on top of gel is stable for 2–5 days.[1] Another source indicates that plasma stored on gel separator barriers show a decrease in glucose concentration from 9% on day 1 to 12% on day 7.[2]

References

1) NCCLS. *Procedures for the handling and processing of blood specimens; Approved Standard—Third Edition.* CLSI document H18-A3. Wayne, PA: Clinical and Laboratory Standards Institute; 2004.

2) Madira WM, Wilcox AH, Barron JL. Storage of plasma in primary plasma separator tubes. *Ann Clin Biochem* 30; 213-214 (1993).

How long can tubes sit before centrifugation?

O ur new doctors are giving me a hard time about letting clot tubes sit before spinning them. The manufacturer recommends the tubes sit for no less than thirty minutes, then spun for fifteen. The doctors want me to spin the tubes 10 minutes after collection. I am very concerned that if I mishandle the blood, the inaccurate results could lead to misdiagnosis, administration of the wrong medication or over/under dosage. I am between a rock and a hard place. Any suggestions?

I t's not unusual for physicians to want results faster, since an estimated 70% of the objective information they receive on their patients' status comes from laboratory tests. However, you are to be commended for upholding the standards for specimen collection and protecting patients from inaccurate results that can come from rushing the process.

There is a myth that clot-activator tubes clot faster, but that's not the case. Your conversation with the tube manufacturer already confirmed that. The purpose of the activator is to facilitate complete clotting, not faster clotting. The end result is a serum sample less likely to have fibrin strands that could interfere with your instrumentation. Keep in mind that a clot-activator tube will gel up quickly and appear to be clotted, but complete clotting still takes up to 30 minutes. Just because the blood doesn't flow when you invert the tube at ten minutes doesn't mean it's clotted.

It's important to know that the risk of premature centrifugation is getting fibrin in the sample, which could gum up the chemistry instrument. If the process is rushed too much, clotting will continue in the serum after centrifugation causing the serum to gel up completely, requiring physical removal of the fibrin in order to get any serum at all. It might help to explain to the physicians that honoring their request can lead to compromised results.

There needs to be a compromise with the physicians, but not with the results. Articulate to the physicians that spinning SST tubes within 10 minutes goes against the tube manufacturer's recommendations, and that doing so puts the lab in legal jeopardy should an inaccurate result be released and acted upon due to fibrin that continues to form in the serum during testing. Have you explored the possibility of conducting your most urgently requested tests on heparinized plasma instead of serum? If you could, then there would be no delay in processing.

Fifteen minutes seems like a long time for centrifugation. Tube manufacturers often have different recommendations for centrifugation times depending on the style of centrifuge. Where 15 minutes might be recommended for a fixed-angle centrifuge, 10 minutes might be adequate in a swivel-head centrifuge. So you might consider investing in a swivel-head centrifuge that spins the tubes at a 90-degree angle to the rotor.

Even though most clot-activator tube manufacturers recommend 30 minutes, most facilities cut the corner without incident. That doesn't make it right, but it shows that you are not the only one pressured for fast turn-around times.

Did You Know...

when citrate tubes for protimes are refrigerated or chilled before testing, cold activation of Factor VII can lead to shortened protime results.

Affects of storage on EDTA specimens

Should EDTA tubes be refrigerated after collection? What about refrigerating the smears? I was told that they should never be refrigerated. We ship our specimens overnight for analysis. Would refrigeration prior to shipping preserve the EDTA specimen? Thanks in advance!

According to Young, platelets decrease by about 8% and hematocrits increase by 7% when stored up to 24 hours at room temperature, but both are stable at refrigerated temps for up to 24 hours. RBCs and WBCs are not affected.[1] Automated differentials are only stable for several hours, depending on the instrument.

We've never heard of any study that measures storage conditions for smears, though. Most labs make the smears when they run the CBC and store them at room temperature.

Reference

1) Young D. *Effects of Preanalytical Variables on Clinical Laboratory Tests.* AACC Press. Washington, DC. 1997.

Chilling serum tubes during transportation

One of our staff has recently begun putting the serum-separator tube in a cup that has a 1/2 inch layer of ice in the bottom. Her rationale is that this will help the blood clot faster so she can then spin the tube. Is there any evidence to support or discourage this practice?

You won't find anything in the literature that supports the practice, and much that contradicts it. The truth is, she's inadvertently guaranteeing that all the potassiums she draws are falsely elevated.

Red cells have 23 times more potassium than the serum or plasma does. What keeps the potassium in the cells is what's known as the sodium-ATPase pump. At refrigerated temperatures, or when your phlebotomist puts her serum tubes on ice, the pump slows and potassium rushes out of the cells into the serum or plasma. Even if kept at room temperature during transportation, the values cannot be considered reliable if more than two hours have passed since collection.

Complete clotting takes up to 30 minutes. Ice won't facilitate it. I'm sure your employee is well intended and only wants to expedite the process for her patients, but attempts to infuse renegade theories into your established procedure should be squelched.

Icing blood gas specimens

Q ur lab's blood gas analyzer requires the blood gas specimen to be transported on watery ice. Is this correct?

A ccording to CLSI document C46, *Blood Gas and pH Analysis and Related Measurements*, plastic syringes should be kept at room temperature, not iced, as long as the blood is analyzed within 30 minutes of collection. Icing specimens is only recommended when transportation and testing are anticipated to take longer than 30 minutes, under which circumstances glass syringes are recommended. You might want to contact the instrument manufacturer to see why they have contradictory recommendations. It may be that the instrument manufacturer's literature doesn't reflect the widespread use of plastic blood gas collection devices.

LDH and storage

We have plasma LDH values that increase over time when stored in gel tubes. In one tube, it went from 173 mEq/L (1 hour post-collection) to 314 mEq/L. In a second patient, it went from 208 mEq/L to 364 mEq/L. Do you think that improper centrifugation and platelet contamination are causing this? The only thing that I can find is that platelet contamination of the plasma can cause increased LDH and potassium. The CLSI guideline states that serum is the specimen of choice but provides no explanation.

Red blood cells have 50 times as much LDH as serum/plasma. Therefore, the least little bit of exposure to RBCs during storage will result in an increase. If the facility uses a fixed-angle centrifuge, the gel can be thick on one side, thin on the other. If there is a break in the gel on the thin side, it could be enough to expose the cells to the plasma. Also, if centrifugation was inadequate, leaving red cells and platelets in the plasma, the LDH in the plasma can increase rapidly as it leaves the red cells.

Make sure you are centrifuging your tubes at the relative centrifugal force (rcf) recommended by the manufacturer for your heparinized gel tube. Don't assume that the rcf is the same as that recommended for your serum tubes. It's probably not.

You also might want to check the package insert of your heparinized gel tubes. Some manufacturers don't recommend storing plasma on their gels.

Phosphorous and preanalytical errors

I am looking for any information on discrepancies with phosphorus results that may be affected by collection or processing techniques.

Serum phosphorous increases when stored in contact with the red cells after three hours at room temperature.[1,2] After separation from the cells, phosphate is stable for four days at room temperature and one week at refrigerated temperatures.[1] Phosphorous does not appear to be posture-sensitive, subject to diurnal variations or affected by hemoconcentration.

References

1) NCCLS. *Procedures for the handling and processing of blood specimens; Approved Standard—third edition.* CLSI document H18-A3. Wayne, PA: Clinical and Laboratory Standards Institute; 2004.

2) Zhang D, Elswick R, Miller W, Bailey J. Effect of serum-clot contact time on clinical chemistry laboratory results. *Clin Chem* 1998;44(6):1325–1333.

Regulations for specimen transport

As our facility does more and more off-site collections, we need a policy for transporting those specimens to our lab. Can you give me some information on this? I've looked at the OSHA web site, but I haven't found anything yet. Thanks for your help.

You might check the US Department of Transportation's web site (www. dot.gov). This agency requires anyone shipping specimens by public carrier to follow its Dangerous Goods Shipping Regulations. Some references that might be helpful to you in applying those regulations to blood specimens include the following:

1) Beckala H. Regulations for packaging and shipping laboratory specimens. *Laboratory Medicine* 1999;30(10):663–7.

2) Tarapchak P. The "wrap" on infectious substances. *Advance for Admin Lab* 2000;10(9):44–7.

3) Mooney B. Wrapped up in shipping specifics. *Advance for Admin Lab* 2002;12(10):72–75.

4) Paxton A. Transporting fluids, blood cultures, and more. *CAP Today* 2004;18(1):34.

5) Rutledge A. Proper shipment of diagnostic, infectious specimens. *Advance for Admin Lab* 2004;14(6):48–53.

6) Appold K. Easy does it: transporting specimens properly. *Advance for Med Lab Prof* June 14, 2004:21–3

Specimen stability in a cooler

Q ow many days is blood good for in a styrofoam cooler for testing? Would the tests results still be accurate after five days? Is there a regulation on this by the FDA? I can't seem to find any information on shipment and proper handling of blood by mail.

A t's not a matter of days, it's a matter of hours. Of the commonly tested analytes, more are unstable after a week than stable. Only sodium and glucose (in sodium fluoride tubes) have stabilities for up to a week at room temperature and uncentrifuged.

Once blood leaves the body, significant and irreversible changes begin to take place. Generally, blood drawn for chemistry and other serum or plasma testing (which requires centrifugation) should be processed within two hours. Chilling serum specimens prior to centrifugation only accelerates the irreversible changes. CBCs are stable for up to 24 hours at room temperature. The Clinical and Laboratory Standards Institute is the organization that establishes specimen storage and handling guidelines and other laboratory standards. If you would like their document on specimen stability, contact them at www.clsi.org and purchase document H18. The FDA doesn't regulate specimen storage recommendations.

Stability of CBC values and sed rates

How long can an EDTA tube sit out before testing and still produce reliable results?

CBCs are good for at least 24 hours refrigerated. At room temperature, most components of a CBC are stable for less than a day. Platelets and hematocrits are the first to change.

During room-temperature storage up to 24 hours, expect platelets to decrease by about 8% and hematocrits to increase by 7%.[1] RBCs and WBCs are not affected for at least three days at room temp or refrigerated.[1,4] Automated differentials are only stable for several hours, depending on the instrument.

Sed rates: 12 hours refrigerated, 4 hours at room temp.[1-4]

References

1) Young D. *Effects of Preanalytical Variables on Clinical Laboratory Tests.* AACC Press. Washington, DC. 1997.

2) NCCLS. *Procedures for the handling and processing of blood specimens; Approved Standard—Third Edition.* CLSI document H18-A3. Wayne, PA: Clinical and Laboratory Standards Institute; 2004.

3) Koepke JA. Update on reticulocyte counting. *Lab Med* 1999;(30):339–343.

4) Gulati G, Hyland L, Kocher W, Schwarting R. Changes in automated complete blood cell count and differential leukocyte count results induced by storage of blood at room temperature. *Arch Pathol Lab Med* 2002;126:336–42.

Thawed specimens

Q ere's the scenario: A specimen is frozen for transport to the testing lab. When the lab thaws the specimen for testing, is vortexing recommended?

A ll serum/plasma specimens should be well mixed prior to testing. Vortexing seems overly aggressive, but there's nothing in the literature that speaks to its effect. A gentle inversion 5–10 times should be sufficient as long as it's completely thawed.

Transporting aPTTs

What is the proper transportation temperature for coagulation studies, particularly aPTTs? We have been transporting them on ice for a long time, but a new phlebotomist is telling us that it's "old school."

According to CLSI, citrate tubes for aPTT testing can be transported at either refrigerated or room temperature.[1] However, transporting protimes on ice is no longer recommended. Chilling such specimens can lead to cold activation of Factor VII, altering protime results.

Temperature is not as much of a concern for aPTTs as time is. Specimens from patients on unfractionated heparin must be centrifuged and separated from the cells within one hour and tested within four hours. Specimens from patients not on heparin must be centrifuged, separated, and tested within four hours. After four hours, aPTTs are not stable unless they've been centrifuged, separated and the plasma frozen at -20°C (two-week stability).

Protimes are much more forgiving. They can be stored at room temperature for up to 24 hours, even uncentrifuged, as long as the stopper has not been removed. Once removed, evaporation takes place, changing the pH and altering test results.

Reference

1) CLSI. *Collection, Transport, and Processing of Blood Specimens for Testing Plasma-Based Coagulation Assays and Molecular Hemostasis Assays; Approved Guideline—Fifth Edition.* CLSI document H21-A5. Wayne, PA: Clinical and Laboratory Standards Institute; 2008.

Transporting protimes

Q e receive protime specimens unspun rather than separated and frozen. Is anyone else doing this?

A ccording to CLSI, protimes are good uncentrifuged for up to 24 hours at room temp or refrigerated as long as the tubes remain unopened. The only reason you might want to spin, separate and freeze the plasma prior to transportation is if you 1) anticipate the addition of an aPTT to the test order; or 2) if the protime will not be tested within 24 hours. Activated partial thromboplastin times (aPTT) are only stable for four hours. Refer to CLSI document H21, *Collection, Transport, and Processing of Blood Specimens for Coagulation Testing Assays and Molecular Hemostasis Assays.* All CLSI documents are available for a fee by calling CLSI at 610-688-0100 or by visiting their web site (www.clsi.org).

Unspun chemistries & coags

Can we ship unspun chemistry and coag specimens to a reference lab overnight and expect accurate results?

You are correct to be concerned about analyte stability in unspun specimens. Unless the lab has data showing longer stabilities, aPTTs and many routine chemistries, especially potassiums, may be compromised. Protimes will be fine, but the literature is full of evidence that many other important analytes are affected when not centrifuged and separated within two hours. Here's what a literature search dug up:

- Protimes are stable unspun at room temperature for 24 hours; seven hours at refrigerated temps. However, aPTTs are only good for four hours at any temperature.[1–3]

- When left in contact with the cells, potassium, glucose, LDH, and ionized calcium are no longer accurate after two hours.[4–5] Refrigerating specimens makes matters worse. However, if glucoses are drawn in fluoride (gray stoppers) they are good for a week.

It's imperative that if you are going to ship overnight, that you centrifuge chemistry specimens within two hours of collection and remove the serum or plasma from the cells. If the tube is a gel tube, the barrier will be adequate for separation and not require further processing. Just remember, not all gel tubes are stable when testing therapeutic drugs. Refer to the limitations, if any, provided by your tube's manufacturer. Gel barriers must be intact and not allow contact between serum and cells.

(cont...)

(Unspun chemistries & coags cont...)

If you are shipping aPTTs, you must centrifuge, separate, and freeze the plasma before shipping. Unseparated, aPTTs are only stable for four hours at any temperature.

Again, if the reference lab has evidence of greater stabilities, these recommendations can be superceded. You might consider requesting such documentation for your peace of mind.

References

1) CLSI. *Collection, Transport, and Processing of Blood Specimens for Testing Plasma-Based Coagulation Assays and Molecular Hemostasis Assays; Approved Guideline—Fifth Edition.* CLSI document H21-A5. Wayne, PA: Clinical and Laboratory Standards Institute; 2008.

2) Reneke J, Etzell J, Leslie S, Ng V, Gottfried E. Prolonged Prothrombin Time and Activated Partial Throboplastin time due to underfilled specimen tubes with 109mmol/L (3.2%) citrate anticoagulant. *Coag Trans Med* 1997;109(6):754–7.

3) Castellone D. How to deliver quality results in coagulation laboratory: commonly asked questions. *Lab Med* 2004;4(35):208–213.

4) NCCLS. *Procedures for the handling and processing of blood specimens; Approved Standard—third edition.* CLSI document H18-A3. Wayne, PA: Clinical and Laboratory Standards Institute; 2004.

5) Young D. *Effects of Preanalytical Variables on Clinical Laboratory Tests.* AACC Press. Washington, DC. 1997.

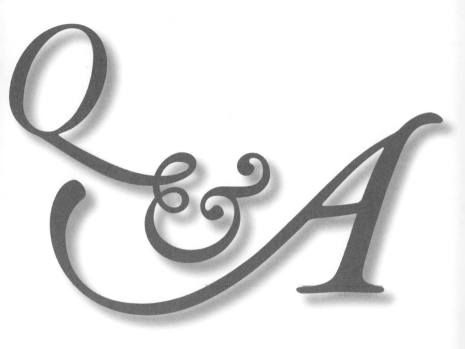

12. Patient Injury & Complications

Patient Injury

Ammonia inhalants

Arterial versus venous blood

Fainting patient and phlebotomy chairs

Fainting patients, reacting to

Forgotten tourniquets

Holding fainting patients for observation

Needle barbs

Patient fainting

Patients waiting for GTT results

Restraining children

Treating suspected nerve injuries

Withdrawing the plunger before inserting the needle

Complications

Iatrogenic anemia in infants

Maximum blood volume

Maximum blood volume/iatrogenic anemia

Maximum volume of blood from fingersticks

Minimum blood volumes

Ammonia inhalants

In a recent lecture, the speaker suggested we don't use an ammonia inhalant as it could trigger an asthmatic attack in susceptible patients. My institution's health nurse and pharmacist have not encountered any safety notices concerning ammonia inhalants, but would appreciate reviewing any studies available on the subject. Could you please guide me to additional information on this subject?

You can cite the CLSI venipuncture standard, which states that the use of ammonia inhalants is not recommended.[1] Several studies support this restriction.[2,3] The risk is that the patient who has lost consciousness, or is feeling faint, may be asthmatic. Because we don't know who is and who isn't asthmatic, it's best to be conservative and avoid ammonia inhalants. The better approach would be to lower the patient's head below his/her heart in combination with a cold compress to the back of the neck or forehead.[1]

References

1) CLSI. *Procedures for the Collection of Diagnostic Blood Specimens by Venipuncture; Approved Standard—Sixth Edition.* CLSI documnet H3-A6. Wayne, PA: Clinical and Laboratory Standards Institute; 2007.

2) Bledsoe BD. This procedure stinks: the hazards of ammonia inhalant use. *JEMS* 2003;28(3)52–3.

3) Herrick R, Herrick S. Allergic reaction to aromatic ammonia inhalant ampule. A case report. *Am J Sports Med* 1983;11(1):28.

Arterial versus venous blood

Ihave been at loggerheads with the physician's assistant in our nursery and with our hematology staff over collecting lavender micro-collection containers from newborns. This morning I found out that the blood they are putting into the tubes is from an arterial stick. The PA says that it is easier to get blood from an arterial stick, so there's no delay in the collection process. Is this an acceptable practice?

Yikes! Performing an arterial stick for routine labs is not appropriate. It subjects the patient to unnecessary risk, and goes against the CLSI standards. There are legal consequences here, so bring your risk manager into the discussion.

Should something go wrong during the arterial stick (a nerve is pierced, inadequate pressure is applied and hemorrhaging occurs that exerts pressure on the nerves leading to permanent injury, etc.) your facility won't have a leg to stand on. All these injuries have occurred in the past from arterial sticks and have led to litigation. If the PA is performing a brachial puncture instead of a radial, it's even worse. Two median nerves pass right along side of the brachial and can easily be pierced. Because infants can't convey the shooting pain sensation that adults can to indicate nerve penetration, the collector may continue to probe.

In the CLSI standard, it explicitly states that arterial sticks are not to be considered a substitute for venipuncture. Common sense should tell us that it's not a substitute for skin punctures, either. Cite the standard. It should give you some muscle to beef up your own blood collection policies.

Additionally, there are clinically significant differences between arterial and venous blood.[1,2] Packed cell volume, lactic acid, ammonia, alcohol, plasma chloride, and glucose all vary. It's a bad idea all around.

References

1) CLSI. *Procedures for the Collection of Arterial Blood Specimens; Approved Standard—Fourth Edition*. CLSI document H11-A4. Wayne, PA: Clinical and Laboratory Standards Institute; 2004.

2) Garza D, Becan-McBride K. *Phlebotomy Handbook*. 7th Ed. Upper Saddle River, NJ Prentice Hall; 2005.

Did You Know...

there are at least 23 documented cases of death due to needle phobia.

Fainting patient and phlebotomy chairs

We recently had a patient fall right out of the chair after he fainted. He fell forward and did some damage to his face and tooth. Our phlebotomy armrest does not lock by design. Are we at risk of a lawsuit? Do phlebotomy chairs need to have a locking armrest?

The CLSI standards state that phlebotomy chairs should have some safety device to prevent fainting patients from falling. Armrests are given as an example. Exactly what mechanism you use is up to you, but a locking arm would certainly qualify. The lack of a locking armrest is not likely to bring liability, but the lack of armrests or other "safety device" could be exploited by an injured patient's attorney.

A second passage also states that a phlebotomy chair should have arms to provide support and prevent falls. Even further in the document, there's a passage that instructs the collector to be prepared to react should the patient lose consciousness. All this indicates some protection should be built into the chair, and the collector should anticipate a loss of consciousness. This means not turning one's back on the patient and always being vigilant to protect the patient from injury should he/she pass out. If the collector left the area or turned his/her back on the patient prior to releasing the patient, that could be effectively argued as operating beneath the standard of care.

Fainting patients — reacting to

We currently have an outpatient lab with a very old donor chair that we use for fainting or ill patients to lie down on. We also have two draw sites not on hospital grounds: one is next to a doctor's office; the other is in an office that does physical therapy. These two draw sites do not have any provisions for ill or fainting patients. What are other facilities doing in these circumstances? I have talked to a few labs and draw sites that have said they put the patient's head between their knees or lay them on the floor. Is this okay to do, or should there be an area where the patient can lie down when they feel ill?

According to CLSI standards, the venipuncture chair should be one that has arm supports to prevent fainting patients from falling. If patients faint, the standards only say to lay the patient flat where it is practical to do so, or lower his/her head and arms if the patient is sitting.

Many outpatient draw stations have a cot or bed for drawing patients who have a history of passing out just in case. Although laying fainted patients on the floor is somewhat uncouth, it can be an appropriate reaction when a cot is not available. As the standard states, lowering the head below the plane of the heart is also acceptable. Whenever considering lowering a patient to the floor, you should seek assistance rather than doing it alone. You can also consider applying a cold compress to the back of the neck or forehead to help revive a patient. Just be careful not to use ammonia inhalants. If the patient happens to be asthmatic, it could trigger respiratory distress.

Forgotten tourniquets

Q I've had three complaints from ICU this past month about phlebotomists leaving tourniquets on their patients. Do you have any suggestions for solving this problem?

You are right to be concerned. Before you discipline your phlebotomy staff, make certain it's not the nursing personnel leaving tourniquets on after surveying sites for IV insertion. If it turns out to be the phlebotomy team, meet with them immediately, explain the potential complications to the patient, state the zero-tolerance policy on forgetting tourniquets, and establish disciplinary consequences. If the nursing staff is culpable, the complications and disciplinary consequences should be addressed by a nurse manager.

Holding fainting patients for observation

I was wondering if there is a standard protocol for handling patients who faint during their specimen collection procedure. I'm looking for advice on immediate care, the amount of time to hold such a patient, physician involvement, and checklists or waivers prior to their dismissal.

There isn't any precedent in the literature as to how long you should hold fainting patients, only that you should be assured they are lucid when they leave your care. But that's more common sense than anything else. It's also up to the facility if you want to refer such patients to a physician before they leave the premises or to have a checklist.

The best approach for immediate care would be to lower the patient's head below their heart in combination with a cold compress to the back of the neck or forehead. There is some concern over the liberal use of ammonia inhalants, so be careful with allowing their use. The risk is that the patient who has lost consciousness or is feeling faint may be asthmatic. If the inhalant is used, it could trigger an asthmatic attack. Because we don't know who is and who isn't asthmatic, it's best to be conservative. The CLSI standards also advise against it.

It's purely up to your facility if you want to have the patient sign a waiver prior to dismissal. It might be a good idea to discuss this with your risk manager. The standards don't address it.

Needle barbs

Q **H**ow common is it for specimen collectors to inspect their needles for barbs before using them? I have not been inspecting them, but our new supervisor insists.

A **A**ccording to the standards, all supplies should be inspected for defects. Most texts suggest inspecting all needles for barbs prior to puncture. In practice, probably less than 5% of collectors actually perform this visual check every time, but it's an important step. In the worst case, barbs can result in a painful puncture and vein trauma resulting in a larger, ragged puncture hole in the skin and vein. As a result, it may take longer for the puncture site to stop bleeding.

Patient fainting

I am a phlebotomy instructor at a local community college doing some research work. Is there any documentation about drawing blood from ambulatory patients sitting on an examination table? I know that this is not appropriate draw procedure, but I am looking for documentation that states it explicitly.

Most textbooks make reference to positioning patients so that they won't be injured if they faint. Although it may be hard to find specific mention of exam tables, you will find supporting evidence in the CLSI venipuncture standard.[1] It states that patients should be seated in chairs suitable for venipuncture and that they should have arms to prevent falls should the patient lose consciousness. Keep in mind, passing out is a risk of phlebotomy that all who collect blood specimens should guard against. Drawing patients who are sitting upright on exam tables does not suggest the collector is anticipating a loss of consciousness.

Reference

1) CLSI. *Procedures for the Collection of Diagnostic Blood Specimens by Venipuncture; Approved Standard—Sixth Edition.* CLSI documnet H3-A6. Wayne, PA: Clinical and Laboratory Standards Institute; 2007.

Patients waiting for GTT results

Our phlebotomy team makes patients wait for the final result on their glucose tolerance test (GTT) to see if it is in an acceptable range. If not, they contact the physician. However, none of the staff know what the "acceptable range" is. Our procedure manual does not require the patient wait. Should it?

Your phlebotomists are doing the right thing, but they don't have all the information they need to fully implement a good policy. To manage the risk, many facilities review the final GTT results prior to letting patients go. Consider this worst-case scenario: a patient completes his GTT and is released. He is a little light-headed and the staff notices that he's not steady on his feet. Unbeknownst to the phlebotomist, his glucose has plunged since the last reading, and he is now in a state of severe hypoglycemia. If the phlebotomist knew the result, the patient could be prevented from getting into his vehicle and losing consciousness while driving.

It's good risk management to assess a final glucose level before releasing the GTT patient, especially in light of clinical signs of hypoglycemia. Your facility should determine what constitutes an acceptable glucose level for the patients before releasing them after a GTT, and have a protocol in place for when it doesn't meet the criteria.

Restraining children

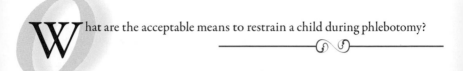

What are the acceptable means to restrain a child during phlebotomy?

Gentle physical restraint is necessary to make sure that the arm to be punctured remains immobile during the venipuncture. Avoid force-fully restraining a child who appears to be calm or only mildly anxious. Kids don't like to be restrained any more than adults do, and a firm, forceful grip can increase their anxiety. It is best to use only as much assistance as is necessary to assure the success of the procedure, and no more.

Regardless of the degree of necessity, restraint should never be applied with a force great enough to cause injury. For outpatients, it is ideal to position the child on the lap of the parent or guardian, who can restrain the free arm of the child while an assistant secures the wrist of the arm to be punctured. For inpatients, or for outpatient situations in which a parent is unable to assist, the patient should lie on a bed or cot with the parent or assistant providing gentle restraint to the legs, the free arm, and the wrist of the arm to be punctured.

Treating suspected nerve injuries

When the patient complains of an electrical, shooting pain, would a warm or cold compress be in order, or should we just inform the nurse in charge of the incident?

⎯⎯⎯⎯⎯⎯⎯⎯⎯⎯⎯⎯⎯⎯⎯⎯

It's beyond the scope of this book to recommend medical treatment. Consider establishing a policy with the input of your medical director or any other qualified physician.

⎯⎯⎯⎯⎯⎯⎯⎯⎯⎯⎯⎯⎯⎯⎯⎯

Withdrawing the plunger before inserting the needle

I have a phlebotomist who uses a technique that I have never seen before. She starts the venipuncture with the syringe plunger pulled back about 1 cc. Isn't there a chance to accidentally introduce air into the vein using this technique?

This technique is patently unacceptable. It sounds contrived and is without support in the literature, the standards, and probably your own procedure manual. You need to squelch this practice before a patient dies of an air embolism.

Iatrogenic anemia in infants

Do you have any suggestions on how to handle a pediatrician who insists that the lab should not be involved in monitoring and advising physicians about the volume of blood we draw from infants? When we notify him his recent order puts his patient over our established limit, he insists on getting all the tests he's ordered and is willing to transfuse if needed to replace blood taken. Should we have a flow chart that documents how much blood has been taken, and let him take it from there?

For the pediatrician to be unconcerned about iatrogenic anemia is disturbing, and puts the facility at risk of operating beneath the standard of care. According to the CLSI standard, document H3-A6, *Procedures for the Collection of Diagnostic Blood Specimens by Venipuncture*, a mechanism to avoid iatrogenic anemia should be in place to monitor the amount of blood drawn from pediatric and critically ill patients.[1] You could establish a policy that requires phlebotomists and other specimen collection personnel to record the volume of blood taken from neonatal patients in their charts, and place the burden of monitoring the volume on the physician. That way, a mechanism would be in place, keeping you in compliance with the standards. You would be managing the laboratory's risk of litigation while placating the physician. However, it still wouldn't protect his infant patients from developing iatrogenic anemia, which is at the heart of the standard. Perhaps by implementing the mechanism, which you are required to do, you would be paving the way for better patient management. You might want to bring your risk manager in on the discussion.

Reference

1) CLSI. *Procedures for the Collection of Diagnostic Blood Specimens by Venipuncture; Approved Standard—Sixth Edition.* CLSI document H3-A6. Wayne, PA: Clinical and Laboratory Standards Institute; 2007.

Maximum blood volume

With the addition of a pediatrician to the staff of our small (70-bed) hospital, we are seeing an increase in the number of pediatric draws. I was able to obtain a chart showing maximum amounts of blood to draw based on the patient's weight, but would like to have more specific guidelines that include the time period in which the maximum amount can be drawn.

There is a chart in the CLSI skin puncture standard (H4) that shows the percentage of a patient's total blood volume that 10 mL constitutes. It's based on the patient's weight and age, but it doesn't make a recommendation as to a maximum amount. It's something your medical staff should consider and establish as policy.

There is another chart out there that signifies the maximum per draw and per hospital stay based on weight. It exists in two textbooks: Garza, Becan-McBride's *Phlebotomy Handbook* and *Applied Phlebotomy* (available online at amazon.com and the usual outlets).

We have a hospitalist who doesn't care how much blood we withdraw from patients. I'm concerned with those who are susceptible to anemia. Many of us reference a chart from the *Applied Phlebotomy Textbook* on maximum blood volumes to collect on patients under 14 years (up to 100 lbs). Do you know of any reference that suggests either maximum volumes or a formula to calculate them on adult patients and/or any patient over 100 lbs?

Your facility should determine the maximum percentage of blood volume to be drawn at one time (or during a set time frame, or both) and develop a chart based on this calculation. Unfortunately, there aren't any references as to what that maximum percentage should be. The CLSI skin puncture standard provides a graph that plots the percentage of a patients' total blood volume that 10 mL constitutes based on the patient's weight and age, but it doesn't make a recommendation as to a maximum amount.

If you consider that donor facilities take out 450 mL of blood from an adult, this constitutes about eight percent total blood volume of a 70 kg adult. This doesn't constitute a recommended maximum, but it's a starting point for a policy that requires the input of your medical director and medical staff.

Facilities should establish a policy with limits that trigger a response when that limit is exceeded. If your medical staff decides that the maximum volume to be drawn is X percent of an infant's total blood volume (or alternatively, X percent of the infant's total circulating red cells), the maximum blood volume to be withdrawn can be easily calculated using the following data:

Total blood volume

Full term newborn: 80–110 mL blood/kg
Premature infant: 115 mL blood/kg
Infants & children: 75–100 mL blood/kg

If a 2.7 kg infant (about 6 pounds) has 80–110 mL blood per kg, then the total blood volume in the infant is between 216–297 mL. If the policy is to remove no more than 7% (arbitrary figure, not a recommendation) of the total blood volume, then multiply 0.07 by the range of 216 to 297 mL and you get a maximum volume of blood to be drawn per draw/day/week/admission (or whatever time frame is established by your facility) of between 15.1 and 20.8 mL.

If you want to consider total RBC volume instead of total blood volume, then you should factor in the average hematocrit value for a newborn (55%). To do so, calculate the total red blood cell volume in the average newborn circulatory system, which approximates 119 mL (216 mL x .55) to 163 mL (297 mL x .55), then set your limit to whatever you decide to be the percentage of RBCs you can safely remove during a given time frame. From there, you can come up with how much whole blood that works out to be.

You could do the same for geriatric populations, but make sure you apply an adult blood volume to the equation instead of one for newborns and infants. You'll also want to adjust their hematocrit downward.

This is just one example of how you might establish a limit, but it's not the only way. Your medical staff needs to agree on a formula and policy after consulting other sources. Double check these figures before you apply them. The best way to comply and silence the hospitalist is to establish a policy that sets limits and triggers a response.

See page 292 for references regarding iatrogenic anemia.

Maximum volume of blood from fingersticks

Do you have any data to suggest what the expected maximum blood volume for a fingerstick should be for both child and adult?

You aren't likely to find any maximum volumes specific for fingersticks in the literature because fingersticks don't typically produce enough blood to cause anemia. If you're performing repeat heelsticks on preemies, however, refer to the same limits your facility has applied to venipunctures for such patients.

Minimum blood volumes

I am concerned with the industry's practice of collecting far more blood for tests than the test actually requires. If a test requires 1 mL of serum, what is the total volume that needs to be collected?

Much has been written on the necessity for minimum draw volumes, but no standards are available. Labs need enough serum for repeat testing; reference labs might need extra in order to send some tests out for confirmation.

Even though many tests can be performed on less than a tenth of a milliliter of serum, much more is required in order for that tenth to be accessible. Assume patients have an average hematocrit of 40% (average between men and women). If a lab requests 1 mL of serum, you should draw about 2 mL of blood. It's important to understand that in 2 mL of blood, not all the serum or plasma is available for testing. Some remains bound in the clot or within the sedimented red cells after centrifugation. Although most chemistry tests can be conducted on a fraction of a milliliter, most automated chemistry instruments require a base amount of serum or plasma from which they can aspirate the required minute amount.

One must also consider the potential for multiple tests on the same sample; repeat testing for confirmation, sending out esoteric tests from the same sample to reference labs, etc. All things considered, drawing five to ten times the amount actually required for testing is not unreasonable to expect a lab to request, especially for tests that require serum or plasma as opposed to whole blood.

(cont...)

(Minimum blood volumes cont...)

Here are some references in the literature on the subject of minimum volumes:

1) McPherson R. Blood sample volumes: emerging trends in clinical practice and laboratory medicine. *Clin Lab Mgmt Rev* Jan/Feb. 2001:3–10.

2) Q&A column. Blood volumes needed for common tests. *Lab Med* 2001;32(4):187–188.

3) Hicks J. Nutrition notes: the need for smaller blood sample sizes. *Adv Admin Lab* 2001;10(7):26.

4) Hicks J. Excessive blood drawing for laboratory tests [Letter]. *N Eng J Med* 1999;340:1690.

5) Zimmerman J, Seneff M, Sun X, Wagner D. et al. Evaluating laboratory usage in the intensive care unit: patient and institutional characteristics that influence frequency of blood sampling. *Crit Care Med* 1997;25(5):737–745.

6) Chernow B, Salem M, Stacey J. Editorial. Blood conservation—a critical care imperative. *Crit Care Med* 1991;19(3):313–314.

7) Peruzzi W, Parker M, Lichtenthal P, Cochran-Zull C, Toth, B. et al. A clinical evaluation of a blood conservation device in medical intensive care unit patients. *Crit Care Med* 1993;21(4):501–506.

8) Lin J. Strauss R, Kulhavy J, Hohnson K, Zimmerman M, et al. Phlebotomy overdraw in the neonatal intensive care nursery. *Pediatrics* 2000;106(2).

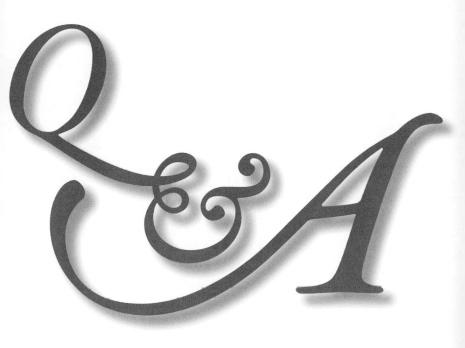

13. Unorthodox Techniques

Bending the needle

Bevel down?

Blood from an arterial line via the "drip method"

Double tourniquet technique

"Harvard" stick

Petroleum jelly to prevent running

Ointment on fingersticks

Reopening a previous heel puncture for more blood

Reopening capillary punctures for more blood

Unorthodox means of applying pressure

Bending the needle

s a nurse and as a phlebotomist in South Africa and now in England, it is common practice to put a slight bend in the needle prior to inserting it into a vein to draw blood. Sterility of the needle is maintained by using the sheath of the needle to bend the needle (bevel facing upwards) as it is uncapped. The bend is more or less half-way down the shaft of the needle and only needs to be slight. About 30 degrees from true. I find the advantages being a less painful, more accurate puncture, decreased likelihood of passing through the vein, the upright orientation of the tube holder allows for an easier exchange, and greater control.

In my experience, there is no risk of hemolysis. However, I have come up against opposition in my technique from phlebotomists in the U.K. I present my case as a request for clarity on whether this practice is acceptable.

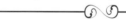

odifying a device post-production is ill-advised on many levels. Manufacturers should be the ones engineering such a modification, not the user. If what you are describing is truly the proverbial better mousetrap, it would already be on the market. By bending the needle, you are using a device against the manufacturer's recommendations. Even though you have experienced patient satisfaction, such an after-market modification is contrived, risky, and should not be conducted. It comes as no surprise that it has aroused passionate resistance.

I would anticipate several concerns:

- If one must remove the sheath to make sure the bevel is up before bending the needle, it surely must incorporate a partial re-sheathing, which risks needle contamination and fingersticks.

- How do you train people to bend the needle to an exact angle every time? If the angle is too great, I would assume the metal would kink and restrict blood flow.

- Such a modification is likely to prevent activation of any safety feature.

(cont...)

(Bending the needle cont...)

If the purpose of bending the needle is to reduce the pain of insertion, the same reduction in pain can be accomplished by making sure the skin is stretched tight prior to puncturing. This practice will not be well received by the medical community in most countries because it involves the use of a needle in a way in which the manufacturer did not intend. It doesn't address a problem that cannot be solved by other means (i.e., stretching the skin). Unorthodox modifications to standardized procedures and equipment with proven performance, like needles, are without justification.

Did You Know...

up to 48% of tube holders
are contaminated with blood after one use.

Bevel down?

Would it ever be appropriate to enter the needle into the vein with the bevel facing down? I want to know if this practice would be appropriate. It seems that this may work in getting into the vein, especially if the needle might be too large for the vein.

This sounds like a home-spun technique; certainly not one supported by the literature. It's difficult to comprehend how an inverted needle orientation would help, i.e., facing upstream instead of downstream. It sounds logical, but at the same time, contrived.

Be careful not to modify such a well-established and standardized procedure as a venipuncture. Once you permit minor deviations, either for yourself or your staff, it won't be long before the procedure morphs so far from the standard that your patients are at risk.

Blood from an arterial line via the "drip method"

We have a physician requesting we implement what he calls the "drip method" when collecting blood via radial or ulnar arterial line draws. I checked our CLSI reference but couldn't find this mentioned. Is there such a thing? Where I might find a reference for it?

By name, it sounds like you're supposed to let the blood drip into the collection tube, potentially exposing the collector to bloodborne pathogens. No text or authoritative treatise describes this technique.

The physician who favors this technique is likely trying to avoid the skewed results that come from hemolysis. That's all well and good, but the potential for exposure to bloodborne pathogens makes the tradeoff unwise. If it's not in your policy to collect blood in this manner—and it shouldn't be—avoid the recommendation. If push comes to shove, bring the laboratory manager and infection control professional in on the discussion.

Double tourniquet technique

I've been asked to research if the practice of using two tourniquets—one above the antecubital and the other at the wrist—for patients who have hard-to-find veins is common. Apparently, some nurses and phlebotomists in our hospital are using this technique for hard draws. I have never heard of this before, but my phlebotomy experience is limited and I am curious to find out if this is a common practice.

This is not a practice; it's malpractice. It's irrational to think that restricting the flow of blood to the antecubital area by tightening a tourniquet around the wrist or forearm is going to make a vein easier to find. It's one of those quirky, homespun modifications that crops up in the literature every now and then that qualifies as "homemade phlebotomy." You won't find any reputable textbook that supports this deviation from the standard. It's a renegade technique that just doesn't belong in anyone's bag of tricks. It's hard telling what other twists to the procedure are being practiced. You'd be well-advised to discipline against such procedural modifications. It's good risk management.

"Harvard" stick

I am the nurse educator in a neonatal intensive-care unit. Most of our nurses perform "Harvard sticks" when unable to obtain blood on our complicated patients. Using the head of the radius and the ulna as landmarks (to form the base of a triangle), you "draw" an inverse triangle on the patient's arm. At the point where the lines intersect, you insert the needle at a 45-degree angle and you're supposed to hit a deep vein.

Most of our nurses were taught the technique by the senior nurses. However, I'm unable to find any written materials on how to teach or standardize this procedure. Would you have any information that you might be willing to share?

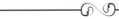

This is one of those techniques that crops up now and then in conversation, but has never appeared in the literature. It seems to be perpetuated in medical schools, and constitutes "homemade phlebotomy." As such, it's equivalent to "blind sticking," which isn't recommended.

Your facility would have little defense if a patient was injured while someone used a procedure that does not have support in the literature, the CLSI standards, any phlebotomy text, and probably not even your own facility's procedure manual. I would highly recommend discouraging this technique from a risk management standpoint.

Petroleum jelly to prevent running

I heard recently that some people use petroleum jelly to smear on a baby's foot to prevent the blood from running away while collecting. Have you heard of this?

This is one of those things people make up because it sounds good or seems right, but you'll never find in a textbook or standards. If blood running off the foot is a problem, then the foot isn't positioned properly. One should position the puncture site fully downward, at its lowest point relative to gravity, so that the blood doesn't have anywhere to run except in the collection tube.

A concern with coating the area with petroleum is that it could interfere with the results. If this technique is to be used, a thorough study of its impact on test results should be conducted in a double-blind study using the appropriate controls for all tests that might be conducted on specimens collected in this manner. It's easier just to position the foot properly. You should discourage this technique.

Ointment on fingersticks

I thought I heard it all until I got a call this afternoon. Many of the fingersticks performed by nurses for CBCs at a local 450-bed hospital come down clotted. One nurse bragged that she never has that problem because she puts a small amount of ointment on the patient's finger just before she performs the stick. The ointment contains vitamins A and D. Have you ever heard of this practice?

Healthcare professionals who were not formally trained are more likely to reinvent the standardized procedure for blood collection. This sounds like the case.

Adding ointments to the skin to facilitate a capillary collection is a new wrinkle (pardon the pun). This might prevent clotting, but I seriously doubt its affects on lab test results have been studied. You should squelch the idea.

Reopening a previous heel puncture for more blood

I was informed that some of our technicians are re-opening an infant's previously poked heel with alcohol, removing the scab, wiping the first drop away, then getting what they need for the test. Is this acceptable?

This technique is not only unacceptable, it's brutal! Besides being painful to the poor infant who is having alcohol rubbed into his/her wound, previously punctured sites that are bruised can yield blood with altered results.

Have your techs stick to the standard, which advises against obtaining blood from the previously punctured site due to accumulated tissue fluid that will contaminate the specimen. Make sure your procedure manual reflects the standard, and then discipline for any policy infractions.

Reopening capillary punctures for more blood

I am the laboratory supervisor of a moderately sized clinic employing a staff of six pediatricians. The nursing supervisor and staff of this peds department have a collective understanding that in the event of a failed capillary puncture, an acceptable recollection technique can include reopening the original puncture with alcohol and recollecting the specimen. In order to educate the department that this is an unacceptable procedure, I need to find written resources detailing the problems that could be encountered when the specimen is recollected in this manner. Would you be willing to help point me to some resources that would be helpful in putting together my presentation?

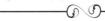

As you know, reopening a previous puncture site to obtain more specimen is unorthodox and ill-advised for a multitude of reasons. This technique, however, is so far "out there" that finding passages in the literature that address this technique is difficult. Not because there is no evidence against it, but because it is inconceivable that the proof in the literature is required to dismiss such an unorthodox practice.

As close as the literature comes to advising against repeat punctures in the same location is the CLSI document H4-A6, *Procedures and Devices for the Collection of Diagnostic Capillary Blood Specimens*. It states that blood must not be obtained from previously punctured sites due to tissue fluid that accumulates and could contaminate the specimen.[1]

Under the general outline for skin punctures, it states that the puncture may be repeated elsewhere if the blood has stopped flowing before the sample is completely collected. At least one textbook reiterates that a different site must be used when performing a second skin puncture.[2]

You might encourage the nurses to prewarm the puncture site for five minutes with a 42-degrees Celsius (or less) warm compress accompanied by gentle massage. Prewarming has been reported to increase the blood flow through the capillary beds seven fold.[1] When sites are properly prewarmed, there is less likelihood that a second puncture will be necessary.

References

1) CLSI. *Procedures and Devices for the Collection of Diagnostic Capillary Blood Specimens; Approved Standard—Sixth Edition.* CLSI document H4-A6. Wayne, PA: Clinical and Laboratory Standards Institute; 2008.

2) Garza D, Becan-McBride K. *Phlebotomy Handbook.* 7th Ed. Upper Saddle River, NJ, Prentice Hall; 2005.

Did You Know...

the fleshy pad of the finger should be used as a
skin puncture site on older children and adults
instead of the sides of the finger to minimize
the potential for bone penetration.

Unorthodox means of applying pressure

C an you tell me the procedure for tightening a tourniquet around the arm and over the puncture site (on top of the cotton ball) as a means of applying pressure to the site to stop the bleeding? We use tourniquets like this for inpatients who are unable to apply pressure themselves. They are left on for a few minutes, then checked by the phlebotomist. Further pressure is applied directly if needed.

T he technique you described is quite unorthodox and not recommended. If the patient is unable to apply adequate pressure, it is the responsibility of the phlebotomist to hold gauze (not cotton) on the site until bleeding has stopped. Using a tourniquet as a substitute for pressure shouldn't be attempted. This technique is certainly without support in the literature.

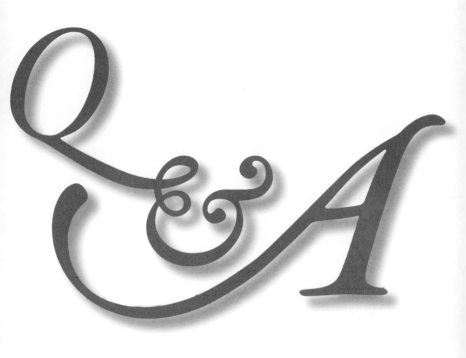

14. Miscellaneous

Allowing addicts to stick themselves

Are platelets activated by vigorous mixing?

CBCs from heparinized syringes

Children in drawing areas

Clotting within a syringe

Clotted EDTA tubes

Contrast media and dyes before venipuncture

Drawing an extra tube

Drawing patients from vehicles

Draws after transfusion

Expelling air from syringes

Fasting defined

Glass coagulation tubes

Hydrating patients with difficult veins

Independent phlebotomist

Jelly beans for glucose tolerance testing

Limits to prewarming

Limits to venipuncture attempts

Making blood smears at the bedside

Mixing gel tubes

Parents/visitors drawing from children/patients

Allowing addicts to stick themselves

We have a drug addict with no veins whatsoever in the usual sites. He wants to insert the needle himself in the vein where he usually injects his drug of choice.

The issue of allowing a drug addict to stick himself scares me and seems to be an open invitation for trouble. I'd like to know the legal angle on that practice.

You are right to be concerned. There's a huge legal liability here. Playing devil's advocate, here's what can happen: The addict is allowed to stick himself. He injures a nerve or nicks an artery and sues for damages (sensing the potential for new way to finance his addiction). The addict's attorney successfully argues that he should not have been allowed to draw his own blood because he has not been trained in the risks of the procedure. To me, it seems to be an open-shut-get-out-the-checkbook kind of case. I'd bring your risk manager in on this and establish a written policy.

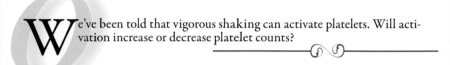

Are platelets activated by vigorous mixing?

We've been told that vigorous shaking can activate platelets. Will activation increase or decrease platelet counts?

You are correct that excessive mixing can activate platelets. Once activated, platelets may clump and cause erroneous readings and instrumentation problems. If not detected, clumped platelets can lead to falsely lower results; clumped platelets are likely to be counted as artifact, white cells, or red blood cells, not platelets. Most modern hematology instruments are capable of flagging platelet results in problem specimens. But don't rely on instrumentation to negate the effect on every specimen.

CBCs from heparinized syringes

When our neonatal nurses draw blood for CBCs, sometimes they perform arterial punctures. They use heparinized syringes and then transfer the blood to EDTA tubes. Are there any adverse consequences to the results when the two anticoagulants are mixed? What do other places do?

There are a couple problems here. First, what you described wreaks havoc with the CBC and needs to be discontinued. One should never mix anticoagulants. Heparin is not a suitable anticoagulant for a CBC, and the practice is likely altering test results. The problem with mixing anticoagulants is that it's impossible for the laboratory to know the specimen contains heparin. Therefore, the lab releases results that may have been compromised without ever knowing the specimen has been adulterated. It's one of the many "hidden" errors that can never be detected by the laboratory and shows up as inaccurate results. Patients may then be treated and managed according to blood levels that may not reflect their actual physiology.

The other problem here is in performing arterial specimens for routine lab work. The myth is that "blood is blood" no matter where you get it, but in actuality, arterial specimens don't compare with venous specimens for many tests. When the laboratory reports a CBC, the lab report includes a normal range for comparison, which is established from venous specimens. So when you submit an arterial specimen for a CBC, the physician is not comparing apples to apples. At the very least, there should be documentation on the report alerting the physician the results are from an arterial specimen.

But simply appending that comment with the result doesn't put you in compliance with the standards. According the venipuncture standard published by the Clinical and Laboratory Standards Institute, arterial punctures are not to be considered as an alternative to venipuncture for difficult draws. So by performing arterial punctures for routine (non blood gas) labs, the nurses are operating beneath the standard of care. This becomes important should the patient be injured during the draw or be treated inappropriately because of results obtained by arterial specimens. So it's a risk management issue as well as a test-result-accuracy issue.

However, if your nurses are drawing blood from an arterial line, that's a bit more understandable. Just make sure you draw the blood gas into the heparinized syringe and the other lab work into a regular sterile syringe. Often routine labs are drawn from arterial lines to save the patient a stick or when there are no other alternatives. As long as the physician knows the results are from arterial blood and not venous, he or she can properly interpret the results. It's the performance of an arterial stick for routine lab work that puts the patient at an increased risk of injury. That's why it's beneath the standard of care to perform an arterial puncture for non-arterial lab tests.

Did You Know...

underfilled EDTA tubes yield a falsely lower hematocrit because red cells shrink when blood is excessively anticoagulated.

Children in drawing areas

What happens when a parent shows up for lab work and insists her child accompanies her? If there is another parent or guardian along, we ask them to wait in the lobby with the child. If not, I put another phlebotomist in the room to watch the child. What are other hospitals doing? Are there references you can refer me to so I can officially address this matter?

Most facilities don't have a formal policy against a parent bringing their child into the outpatient drawing area. Nor do they assign another phlebotomist to watch the child. The child remains under the supervision of the parent. But there are several things to be concerned about here. Sharps containers should be well out of reach of all children. During the venipuncture, there's always the potential for the child to reach for the needle while it's going into the mother's arm. Mothers need to make sure they instruct their child not to interfere or to explore the supplies and equipment of the drawing area.

Arranging the area so that things are out of reach is an added precaution and good risk management. One final thought: there may be some benefit to having a child witness the collection. If the child sees how simple the procedure is and that it brought no discomfort to the parent, they are likely not to be apprehensive when they have to have their own blood drawn.

Further reading

1) Harty-Golder B. Who should supervise children in a patient waiting area? *MLO* 2002;34(9):24–25.

Clotting within a syringe

When a specimen is collected into a syringe from a vascular-access device like a central line, how much time do you have before you should transfer the blood from the syringe to an evacuated tube? How quickly will the specimen clot as it sits in the syringe? We use plastic syringes and plastic evacuated tubes. ———————————————

There is no set limit, but you should transfer blood from a syringe into tubes as soon as possible. Although the syringes, being made of plastic, aren't going to facilitate clotting like a glass tube does, it will still eventually clot. Setting the syringe down for any period of time is not wise, nor in the best interest of specimen integrity.

In one facility, an ER nurse drew blood into a syringe, set it aside to manage the IV, then evacuated the blood into the tubes after some time had passed. The EDTA tube produced a hemoglobin of 5.4 mg/dl, which prompted an immediate crossmatch. Before transfusing, the physician ordered another CBC just to be sure. The second hemoglobin measured was 11.8 mg/dl. The lab speculated that there was sufficient clotting in the syringe to cause the erroneous initial result.

Clotted EDTA tubes

We are currently seeing an increased incidence in clotted EDTA samples. Our pediatric clinicians are very upset with the delays and re-sticks. I believe the cause of this increase is two-fold; the tube manufacturer has a back order on the collection tubes we use for pediatric samples, and we have not done a great job of educating hospital staff members who are collecting our blood samples. How do you recommend we educate our staff on mixing specimens?

Clotting is a common problem, and the most common reason for hematology specimen rejection. Make sure you constantly reinforce inverting specimens immediately. Too often an "inversion" is just a quick back and forth with the hand. Make sure your collectors slow down the process and let the air bubble within travels the entire length of the tube before bringing it back upright. That's one inversion. Most tube manufacturers recommend 5–10 inversions for EDTA tubes. If you stressed slower, more deliberate inversions, you'd have fewer rejected specimens. But you have to be diligent and thorough in your reminders.

Contrast media and dyes before venipuncture

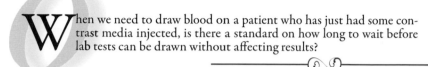

When we need to draw blood on a patient who has just had some contrast media injected, is there a standard on how long to wait before lab tests can be drawn without affecting results?

Fluorescein dye has been reported to interfere with creatinine, cortisol and digoxin measurements.[1] The text cites the following article:

Elin R, Bloom J, Herman D, et al. Interference by intravenous fluorescein with laboratory tests. *Clin Chem* 1989;35(6):1159.

A second reference book, which summarizes the literature on preanalytical errors, points to a study that shows fluorescein increases bilirubin, creatinine, digoxin (on the Abbott TDx), urine protein, and a retic counts. It's listed as decreasing ionized calcium and urine creatinine.[2] Iodine as a contrast media has been shown to cause spurious bicarbonate and chloride results due to analytical interference of the absorbed iodine during a cystogram.[3] Another study showed iodine in the iodinated contrast agent Ioxaglate causes a dose-dependent prolongation of thrombin time, thrombin coagulase time, partial thromboplastin time and calcium thromboplastin time.[4] Iodinated contrast media alters RBC morphology.[5,6]

As a general rule, the more time that passes, the better, but that's based on common sense more than anything else. At the very least, specimens should be labeled as being drawn after the infusion of radiologic dyes and a notation accompanying the test result. Stating the time of the infusion and the name of the dye or contrast media would help interpret test results properly.

References

1) Garza D, Becan-McBride K. *Phlebotomy Handbook*. 7th Ed. Upper Saddle River, NJ Prentice Hall; 2005.

(cont...)

(Contrast media and dyes before venipuncture cont...)

2) Young D. *Effects of Preanalytical Variables on Clinical Laboratory Tests*. AACC Press. Washington, DC. 1997.

3) Abdel-Wareth LO, Lirenman DS, Halstead AC, McLellan D, Carleton BC. Spurious rise in total carbon dioxide and chloride with negative anion gap after cystogram. *Pediatr Nephrol* 1995;9(3):348–50.

4) Schulze B, Beyer HK, Hanstein U. The in-vitro-effects of loxaglate (Hexabrix) on coagulation, fibrinolysis and complement system (author's transl)(Article in German) *Rofo* 1981 May;134(5):566–70.

5) Aspelin P, Stöhr-Liessen M, Almén T. Effect of iohexol on human erythrocytes. Changes of red cell morphology in vitro. *Acta Radiol Suppl* 1980;362:117–22.

6) Man EB. A note about iodine-containing contrast media and the interference of teridax for cholangiograms in evaluation of thyroid function by measurement of serum iodine. *Am J Roentgenol Radium Ther Nucl Med* 1960;83:497–500.

Did You Know...

one study showed that up to 16 percent
of arm bracelets in some facilities have
erroneous information.

Drawing an extra tube

A t our facility, green tops are usually drawn for chemistries during morning rounds. Are there any problems with drawing an extra red top tube on in-patients who may get lab tests ordered later that require serum? This would save the patient from being stuck a second time. Are there any legal or ethical issues involved with this practice?

I t seems that such a practice would only be problematic if the patient is already anemic, neonatal, or has some other disorder that drawing an additional specimen would make risky. However, drawing an extra tube on every patient is probably excessive and not justified by your frequency of add-on tests. Consider this practice on a case-by-case basis. When add-ons are likely, it seems that drawing an extra tube could be in the patient's best interest. Above all, follow facility policy.

Drawing patients from vehicles

O ur outpatient department wants to consider drawing patients sitting in their car. Our previous insurance carrier had told us not to take the risk, recommending instead that our home health department should collect these types of patients. Our current insurance carrier admitted that none of their 75 client hospitals are currently collecting in private vehicles, but they didn't advise against the practice. If other hospitals are doing this, what written policies do they have to cover themselves? Do you have an opinion about collecting blood samples in private vehicles?

F or the record, there are no laws addressing this that we know of; nor is drawing patients from their vehicle addressed in any of the standards or textbooks. It would be surprising if the insurance carrier's other 75 hospitals don't occasionally draw patients in their vehicles. Your contact at the insurance agency is probably just not aware of the practice. The service is probably offered on an as-needed basis in most facilities.

It may be good customer service, but there are risks. Your facility may consider the courtesy only for those patients who can't otherwise walk or be assisted to the draw station. It would be wise to establish that the courtesy will only be provided if the patient is a passenger, not the driver. When drawing patients who ambulate to the drawing room, the collector can observe for the signs of an imminent loss of consciousness. However, when a patient is drawn while sitting in a vehicle, these observations are compromised.

If the passenger passes out, the risk of injury is minimal. If a driver passes out, the risk is significant for the patient and others on the road. Your risk manager should be consulted on the issue. He/she will probably concur.

Draws after transfusion

How long should I wait after a blood transfusion before drawing blood for testing?

Drawing blood during/after a transfusion is a function of what is being drawn. When a physician orders a post-transfusion blood count, the objective is to obtain a homogeneous mixture of patient and donor blood. This is difficult when the patient is receiving blood because of an acute hemorrhage, because homogeneity will not occur until the hemorrhaging has been arrested. The time it takes post-transfusion to achieve homogeneity depends on a multitude of variables including the condition of the patient's heart, kidneys, and circulatory system, the patient's pre-transfusion blood volume, and the age and volume of the transfused cells. Nevertheless, the beneficial effect of an infusion is often vital information to the physician.

Cell counts drawn during a transfusion provide little useful information except in cases where the patient's condition is changing rapidly. It is conceivable that accurate cell counts can be obtained immediately after transfusion.[1] However, delaying the draw for an hour after the transfusion may provide more accurate results if time permits. Such determinations should be made by the physician on a case-by-case basis.

When drawing post-transfusion blood for chemistry assays, the donor blood temporarily raises the level of some analytes for prolonged periods. A significant percentage of the cells in a donor unit may be hemolyzed during storage. Therefore, specimens drawn after transfusion can show elevated levels of plasma hemoglobin, potassium, LD, and serum iron.[2,3] These levels can remain elevated up to 24 hours depending on the patient's kidney function and other variables.

(cont...)

(Draws after transfusion cont...)

CLSI doesn't address post-transfusion cell counts in its venipuncture standard, but the document is quite detailed on the proper procedure for drawing blood from a patient receiving IV fluids of any kind, including donor blood.[4] In one passage, CLSI states that draws from the same arm as an infusion should be avoided if at all possible. Although drawing above an active IV is discouraged in many documents,[4-6] when unavoidable CLSI suggests collectors have the IV shut off for two minutes prior to the puncture, tighten the tourniquet, and perform the puncture as usual. Some authors and studies suggest discarding the first 3-10cc of blood.[7-9] All blood drawn from the same arm as an IV infusion should be documented as such.[4]

References

1) McBride K, Eisenbrey A, Haraden L. Venipuncture after transfusion. *Adv Med Lab Prof* January 25, 1999:4.

2) Narayanan S. The preanalytic phase an important component of laboratory testing. *Am J Clin Pathol* 2000;113:429–452.

3) Mayhre B. Iron values after transfusion. Tips on Specimen Collection. *Medical Economics* Montvale, NJ. 1997.

4) CLSI. *Procedures for the Collection of Diagnostic Blood Specimens by Venipuncture; Approved Standard—Sixth Edition.* CLSI document H3-A6. Wayne, PA: Clinical and Laboratory Standards Institute; 2007.

5) Watson R, O'Kell R, Joyce J. Data regarding blood drawing sites in patients receiving intravenous fluids. *Am J Clin Pathol* 1983;79(1):119–121.

6) Read D, Viera H, Arkin C. Effect of drawing blood specimens proximal to an in-place but discontinued intravenous solution. *Am J Clin Pathol* 1988;90(6):702–706.

7) Garza D, Becan-McBride K. *Phlebotomy Handbook.* 7th Ed. Upper Saddle River, NJ: Prentice Hall; 2005.

8) Dale J. Preanalytic variables in laboratory testing. *Lab Med* 1998;29(9):540–545.

9) Mohler M, Sato Y, Bobick K, Wise L. The reliability of blood sampling from peripheral intravenous infusion lines. *Jrnl of Intravenous Nurs* 1998;21(4):209.

Expelling air from syringes

I am a fairly new phlebotomist, and there is a bit of discrepancy regarding syringe draws where I work. Some people say the syringe should be pumped to "loosen up" the plunger; others say that to do so introduces air into the chamber and potentially contaminates the syringe. Which is correct?

If you look closely at a new syringe, you will notice that the plunger is not fully depressed to the hub. The plunger is "sealed." Before using, the seal needs to be broken by pulling back and then pushing it forward all the way to the hub to fully expel all the air in the barrel. The potential for specimen contamination with the air that enters the barrel during this process is negligible. Just make sure you don't contaminate the tip of the syringe while attaching the needle.

Fasting defined

My patients are told by their physicians to fast for 12 hours and to ingest nothing except water. Other physicians tell them they can have black coffee or tea. Still others just tell them not to ingest anything after midnight. I have also heard that a diabetic should never fast, but then I hear nurses tell patients a 10-hour fast is fine! What's the standard definition of "fasting"?

Fasting is defined as a 10–12 hour overnight dietary restriction of everything except water and medications. For lipids, studies show a daytime fast is acceptable. But for glucose, it must be overnight. As for coffee and tea, physicians often allow patients this luxury as a gesture of compassion. Studies are inconclusive as to whether or not coffee or tea affects fasting lipid levels. Some studies show significant changes, some show none. If you know your patient has had coffee during a fast, include that information on the report with the results so the physician can interpret them properly.

The claim that diabetics shouldn't fast seems somewhat odd. Everybody, diabetic or not, fasts to a certain extent while they sleep. If their glucose is under control, an overnight fast shouldn't be a problem.

Glass coagulation tubes

S ome reps are telling us that glass is the "gold standard" for coag tubes. I think it's outdated information. What's the bottom line?

────────────○○ ○○────────────

T he consensus among coagulation authorities is that glass syringes and tubes must be avoided for coagulation studies since glass activates clotting factors. The early work on glass activation of coagulation factors is found in a paper by Harvey Gralnick way back two decades ago.[1] This was related to glass syringes and/or collection tubes that were stored in ice in order to preserve labile coagulation factors, which, of course, were not well preserved. Jean Thompson wrote a very detailed chapter in *Laboratory Hematology* titled "Specimen Collection for Blood Coagulation Testing" (JA Koepke, Editor. Churchill Livingstone. 1984). This chapter recounts much of the work that has been done to ensure adequate specimens for testing. In recent years, various manufacturers have developed plastic tubes and coatings designed to avoid contact activation. Plastic tubes and/or various coatings are state of the art now.

The surface of collection tubes that activate the coagulation cascades, like glass, may significantly alter test results. According to CLSI guidelines, all surfaces that blood for coagulation testing comes in contact with should be "non-wettable" to deter activation.[2] Studies have shown that plastic coagulation tubes perform equivalently to glass coagulation tubes for routine coagulation studies, i.e., the differences are clinically insignificant.[3,4]

References

1) Gralnick, HR & Palmer, R. *Cold-induced contact surface activation of the prothrombin time in whole blood. Report of the Subcommittee on Standardization of Prothrombin Time.* International Committee on Thrombosis & Haemostasis, Toronto, 1981.

(cont...)

(Glass coagulation tubes cont...)

2) CLSI. *Collection, Transport, and Processing of Blood Specimens for Testing Plasma-Based Coagulation Assays and Molecular Hemostasis Assays; Approved Guideline—Fifth Edition.* CLSI document H21-A5. Wayne, PA: Clinical and Laboratory Standards Institute; 2008.

3) Flanders B, Crist R, Rodgers G. A comparison of blood collection in glass versus plastic Vacutainers on results of esoteric coagulation assays. *Lab Med* 2003;10(34):732–5.

4) Barclay L. Coagulation testing not affected by plastic vs glass. *Medscape Medical News* www.medscape.com/viewarticle/494703?src=mp. Accessed 5/16/08.

Did You Know...

retics are only stable for 6 hours at room temperature.

Hydrating patients with difficult veins

I was taught in phlebotomy school that if a fasting patient has not had any water, they may be dehydrated and impossible to draw. Is this true?

⎯⎯⎯⎯⎯ ᥫ ᥫ ⎯⎯⎯⎯⎯

The theory that drinking water makes it easier to find veins in dehydrated patients may be valid. Although it has never been tested and proven, many veteran phlebotomists claim it works. It makes sense that it would.

⎯⎯⎯⎯⎯ ᥫ ᥫ ⎯⎯⎯⎯⎯

Independent phlebotomist

I'm increasingly frustrated with my work. I want to try to find a way to be a self-employed contractor in phlebotomy somehow. Do you know of any phlebotomy companies that work like homecare agencies? I don't want to work for anyone, but me! Any ideas?

You have several options. There are some mobile phlebotomy services that have been started by phlebotomists like you who wanted to be self-employed. You might also consider working as an independent contractor for insurance companies. They hire phlebotomists, or contract with companies that hire phlebotomists, to perform insurance examinations including blood pressure checks, taking applications, and collecting blood and urine samples. The pay is good. Two major companies that hire contract phlebotomists are L&L Paramedical and Portamedic. If you are in a major metropolitan area, your local insurance industry is likely served by one or the other, or both.

Jelly beans for glucose tolerance testing

W hen screening for gestational diabetes mellitus in pregnant patients who can't tolerate the beverage, are there any substitutes for the loading dose of glucose? Someone suggested jellybeans as an alternative to the 50-gram glucose beverage. Is there a standard that specifies the brand, number, and concentration of each bean? It seems dangerous to assume all brands/types of jellybeans would work equally well.

T wo articles discuss jellybeans as a substitute for a glucose beverage. Their abstracts are both available on PubMed at www.pubmed.com.

One of them used 28 jellybeans as a substitute for 50 grams of glucose. (They calculated that 28 beans equated to 50 grams of a simple carbohydrate.) They found no significant difference between the control group (glucose beverage) and the study group.[1]

The second study compared the use of 18 jelly beans versus 50 grams of glucose. The abstract is full of stats that aren't summarized well, but the authors conclude, "jelly beans may serve as an alternative to a cola beverage containing 50 grams of glucose."[2] Neither study abstracts stated the brand of jellybean. Perhaps the full article does. They're referenced below.

References

1) Lamar M, Kuehl T, Cooney A, Gayle L, Holleman S, Allen S. Jelly beans as an alternative to a fifty-gram glucose beverage for gestational diabetes screening. *Am J Obstet Gynecol* 1999;181(5, pt. 1):1154–7.

2) Boyd K, Ross E, Sherman S. Jelly beans as an alternative to a cola beverage containing fifty grams of glucose. *Am J Obstet Gynecol* 1995;173(6):1889–92.

Limits to prewarming

One of our phlebotomists has her patients put their hands under hot water prior to a venipuncture to the back of their hands. We think the extreme temperature is why we see slight hemolysis and unexplained critical protimes. Our suggestion is to use the heel warmers with a defined temperature range or towels soaked in "warm water" as a second choice. Do you have an opinion on this?

Prewarming sites for fingersticks and venipunctures can increase the flow of blood through the area dramatically, increasing the likelihood of a successful puncture. However, the maximum temperature should be 42-degrees Celsius. Should the water be so hot that it burns a patient, there would be liability issues. Prewarming has not been reported to cause hemolysis or altered test results, however.

Limits to venipuncture attempts

Q How many times can a person attempt to draw blood on the same patient?

A ccording to the standards, attempting a venipuncture more than twice is not advisable. The requirement is to seek the assistance of another person if possible, or notify the physician. As written, the standard indicates that the collector who misses twice must at least make an attempt to find someone else skilled in the procedure to draw the patient. If no on can be located, it may be acceptable for the same collector to try beyond two attempts, providing it is permitted by your facility's policy. There is nothing written in the standards or elsewhere that limits how many different individuals can attempt to draw the same patient.

Making blood smears at the bedside

I am a phlebotomist at a small hospital lab. It's hard to believe in this day and age, but I'm required to do blood smears at the patient's bedside. That means, if the procedure calls for a fingerstick, I have to squeeze a drop from the finger onto a couple of slides, and play with it there in front of the patient. If it's a venipuncture, I have to use a syringe and not activate the safety device until I squeeze blood onto the slides. Surely there's an OSHA or other standard out there I can wave in front of my supervisor to stop this, isn't there?

You are right. This is a little hard to fathom. Unless there's more to the story, slides can be made from the EDTA tube when the specimen arrives in the hematology department. The Bloodborne Pathogens Standard states "engineering and work practice controls shall be used to eliminate or minimize employee exposure." It defines a work practice control to be "controls that reduce the likelihood of exposure by altering the manner in which a task is performed."

Because smears can be made directly from the EDTA tube without the risk of a needlestick, the practice you described could subject the facility to a fine and citation.

In the latest OSHA Compliance Directive, which is a document that tells inspectors how to interpret the standard, "If a combination of engineering and work practice controls used by the employer does not eliminate or minimize exposure, the employer shall be cited for failing to use engineering and work practice controls."

Bring this to the attention of your management and infection control nurse tactfully. If they have a good reason why it's better than making slides from the EDTA tube, listen with an open mind. It may be legitimate. If so, protect yourself by activating the safety feature of the needle, removing it from the syringe and discarding it. Apply a drop to the slide from the hub of the syringe, then apply a safety transfer device to fill the tubes required.

But you should not have to subject yourself to this antiquated process without a good reason. Without one, coupled with their failure to remove the hazardous practice, a call to OSHA may be your last resort.

You can access the Bloodborne Pathogens Standard and the Compliance Directive at: http://www.osha.gov.

Did You Know...

59% of all transfusion errors occur because of improper patient identification either at the time of specimen collection or at the time of transfusion.

Mixing gel tubes

Is the phlebotomist supposed to invert a clot activator tube to insure that the blood has mixed with the clot activator? My lab manager disagrees with this and said that she is boss and that I am not to do this. The package insert demonstrates mixing the tubes. What do I do? Follow the manufacturer or the lab manager?

You're in a pickle, here. You are correct that even clot activator tubes need to be mixed. Sounds like there are more undercurrents to this disagreement than what's evident on the surface. You are clearly in the right, but the unasked question is why does your manager insist on exerting her authority in this way? "Because I said so" is fine when the directive has a basis, but the case you described sounds like there's more at work here than just a disagreement on mixing red tops.

In the interest of getting along, see if you can sit down with the boss and ask her what's really driving this conflict. Perhaps it's the way you pleaded your case or some unresolved issues from long ago, who knows. But it's important you both get a chance to clear the air in an open, civilized, manner.

Parents/visitors drawing from children/patients

Do you know of any policy/rules concerning a parent drawing their child's blood? A friend at a nearby hospital had a pediatric patient that the phlebotomist missed and the parent (who was a nurse) wanted to draw her child's blood.

This is a risk management nightmare. Allowing visitors or parents not employed by the facility to draw blood on their loved ones is really sticking your neck out.

It's impossible to know the extent of their training, their grasp of the standards, or their competency. If they drew the blood in a manner in which you knew the results could be compromised—for example, in the wrong order of draw or with the tourniquet left on too long—would you still accept the specimen? What if they injured the patient? When you allow an outsider to perform a function that is normally provided by your own trained, supervised, and regularly evaluated staff, it has the potential to become a legal nightmare.

I understand that parents skilled in phlebotomy want to minimize the trauma to their child or loved one by doing it themselves, but the facility may be held responsible for any injury or complications. Have a conversation with your risk manager and draft a policy if you need one. The issue will likely come up again eventually, and it's nice for you to be able to simply say "it's against facility policy."

Phlebotomists diagnosing patients

I recently had a physician complain because my staff did not recognize the signs of cyanosis and draw extra tubes of blood. It turned out the patient had a hematocrit of 70! I can't find any references on the Internet about phlebotomy and the cyanotic patient. Can you help?

I'm afraid the physician is expecting more from your staff than he/she has a right to. You won't find any references to cyanosis and phlebotomy because phlebotomists are not trained to clinically evaluate patients and draw the appropriate tubes and volumes of blood. It's unrealistic to expect them to. The physician should be reminded that phlebotomists are not trained to diagnose, and have to rely on the physician to be on top of the patient's condition. I think the expectation is way out of line and inappropriate.

If phlebotomists are to diagnose conditions and draw the appropriate specimens on cyanotic patients, are they also to take it upon themselves to draw blood gases on all patients who are short of breath? This is a can of worms that's best left unopened.

Phlebotomists having seizures

If a phlebotomist were to have a seizure while performing a venipuncture, what, if any, precautions would need to be in place to ensure the patient's well-being?

Ideally, phlebotomists prone to seizures wouldn't be put in patient situations that could be potentially harmful to the patient. Rather, they would be moved into specimen processing roles where a seizure is less likely to affect a patient during the procedure. It's good risk management for phlebotomists prone to seizures to be moved into positions that don't put the patient at risk. From a liability standpoint, a jury wouldn't look favorably on a healthcare facility that allowed such employees to be in a position where they could have a seizure while the needle is in the patient's arm.

Posture and osmolality

During a lecture today about osmolality it was mentioned the position of the patient is a factor. Do you have a reference I could check to confirm this?

The study referenced below showed that serum osmolality is higher when the patient is standing than when sitting (291 mosmol/kg versus 287). The reference is a bit dated, but it's the only one we're aware of.

Reference

1) Itoh Y, Kawai T. Diurnal and postural variation in serum a1-microglobulin in normal individuals. *Clin Chem Acta* 1991;201:123–128.

Posture sensitive analytes

I'm a staff nurse at a health center wanting to educate my unit on correct blood drawing technique, particularly with regard to coagulation studies. With postural changes from lying to sitting, you get a temporary decrease in plasma volume. Will this temporarily increase or decrease the hematocrit? Will it temporarily prolong or shorten the aPTT and INR?

You are correct that a change in posture from recumbent to upright temporarily decreases plasma volume. Many analytes are affected, including coagulation proteins. In order to understand why, let's summarize what happens in vivo when the patient changes posture.

When a patient goes from lying down to upright, there's a temporary loss in blood volume, especially above the heart. The brain senses the change in orientation and releases the hormones that increase blood pressure and, subsequently, blood volume. So, as you astutely observed, blood volume decreases initially, then increases to a point of over-compensation when the body increases blood pressure as a natural reaction to keep the brain, suddenly elevated, fed with oxygenated blood.

Because of the suddenly higher blood volume and intravascular pressure, the capillary walls become porous, allowing water and smaller compounds to efflux into the tissue. Anything too large to pass through the capillary walls (i.e., cells, large molecular weight compounds and those bound to protein) stays in the circulating bloodstream. As a result, their concentrations temporarily increase. We know this as hemoconcentration. (A nice graphic animation of this phenomenon is in the "Preventing Preanalytical Errors" video. Visit www.phlebotomy.com/video.html for more information.)

Hematocrits, cellular indices, and other analytes can falsely increase when a patient changes from recumbent to upright. Not all change to a clinically significant degree, however. It's best to refer to your facility's test requirements and honor posture considerations where specified.

Pouring off blood from one tube to another

We continue to have a problem with a phlebotomist who pours blood from one type of tube into another. One nightmare we experienced was when she poured a sample collected in a lavender top tube into an SST tube for a comprehensive profile. The phlebotomy programs and training manuals clearly define the importance of the order of draw, but in the real world when a phlebotomist is trying to recover from a short draw, short cuts often occur. Do you have any articles or available literature regarding the integrity of a sample that is poured from one collection tube into another?

Having to provide documentation that it's improper to pour the contents of one tube into another tube is like having to prove you shouldn't draw from the jugular. Some things don't require a study.

No text comes out and states you shouldn't do this. But it's one of those things that should be so blatantly obvious that it wouldn't even be conceived by those who are properly trained. This is nothing more than a homespun solution that reflects a lack of understanding of specimen integrity. Clearly the phlebotomist needs more comprehensive training.

Preassembling collection devices

We have phlebotomists who want to save time by taking the syringe and needle out of their packaging and assembling them before going to the patient's room. They tell me this "speeds up" the collection process. I am not in favor of that because of infection control, but I can't find anything to support me. Can you provide any help?

The argument that preassembly "speeds up" the collection process is fallacy. The time saved might amount to four seconds per patient. If your phlebotomists are in that much of a hurry, they shouldn't be drawing blood. Heaven only knows the other shortcuts they're taking for expediency.

In the CLSI venipuncture standard, the sequence of events lists assembling equipment as step number 4, which comes after approaching and identifying the patient. So, although the standard doesn't come right out and say "Do not assemble equipment in advance," it can be inferred by the position of the assembly step in the recommended sequence. That should be all the evidence you need to reorganize your phlebotomists' priorities. Just make sure your procedure manual reflects the standards in this regard, and you will have even more leverage.

It's not only a good policy from an infection control standpoint, but patients want to see the devices being used on them assembled before their eyes. It assures them the collector is not using the same needle used on the last patient. If these reasons aren't good enough, then try "Because I said so." Make it part of your written policy, then you can discipline against infractions.

If your facility allows needles and tube holders to be preassembled, what guarantee does the staff have that the needle on their tray has never been used before? If phlebotomists swap trays, they are putting a lot of trust in each other that someone else didn't recap a used needle and return it to the tray. Stranger things have happened.

Racist patients

How should I handle this scenario: a phlebotomist goes into a patient's room, and the patient refuses to allow the phlebotomist to draw his blood because of the phlebotomist's race? The phlebotomist feels the employer should do something. What should be done?

This is an emotionally explosive situation. The easy way out would be to allow the patient's racism to dictate the running of the hospital. However, it's important to keep in mind that doing what's right is rarely the easy option. Placating racism will only reinforce it.

Those subjected to racism like this need to avoid the knee-jerk reaction, which would be to become enraged and offended. A more professional approach would be to convey the facility's policy of not hiring or managing employees according to race, and that it doesn't entertain racist-based requests from patients (assuming, of course, that the employer has and supports such policies).

More than likely, this strategy won't dissuade the racist patient, but it will establish the facility's policy. Such a policy should be established after consulting with the facility's risk manager and legal counsel.

Sexism in the workplace

I have been trying for months to find work and I always get denied for use-less reasons like "not enough experience" or some other lame excuse that I cannot possibly change as a recent grad. I realize that not too many men are working in this industry; that does not bother me. But nobody ever told me how sexist this field is toward men. I am so fed up that I have been applying out of the country. What should I do to report this, or is this just part of the game?

While it's true the profession is predominantly women, many men work in the field. With the high turnover rate and the low availabil-ity of qualified applicants, most managers are happy to hire qualified applicants of either gender. When you apply, stress your best qualities and make sure you don't come across as threatening. Take a hard look at your qualities and demeanor to see if there could be some other underlying characteristic that is turning off potential employers. Do you dress appropriately for your interviews? Do you present yourself in a positive manner? Do you express your expertise adequately? Are you overly aggressive? There are many red flags that cause managers to shun applicants. Be careful that you are not jumping to the wrong conclusion about gender bias being the cause.

Therapeutic phlebotomy and immunity

I have a patient who has frequent phlebotomies due to hemochromatosis. He is concerned that continually withdrawing his blood may affect his immunity to the common cold and the flu. What advice should I give him?

Your patient needn't be concerned about depleting his immunity. The body is a beautiful and complex system, and makes the necessary adjustments when the he has blood removed.

The body reacts to infections in two ways: a cellular response (white blood cells) and an immune response (antibodies), both of which are triggered by an invasion from something foreign (bacteria, virus, etc.). The immediate response to an infection is the cellular response, which rises up from the bone marrow and lymph nodes (to a lesser extent, from the circulatory system) to defend the body. So even if the patient has been phlebotomized for a unit of blood, the cellular response is barely compromised. In fact, in response to the depletion in circulating white blood cells, the bone marrow and lymph nodes go into accelerated production to replace the lost cells that patrol the circulatory system and tissue for infection. Perhaps the patient's physician could reinforce this.

Training arms

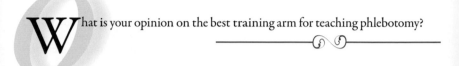

What is your opinion on the best training arm for teaching phlebotomy?

At the Center for Phlebotomy Education, we have tried many models over the years. The one that provides the most life-like experience is the Advanced Venipuncture Training Aid. That's why it's the only one we offer in our catalog. We have tried the arms that are anatomical in appearance, but find that, while they look realistic, they don't feel natural when palpating or inserting a needle. Most have an unnatural air space between the simulated skin and the vein. If your student misses the vein, he/she gets air in the tube and has to apply tube after tube until the vein is accessed. That's not what happens in real patients. It's just not a life-like experience.

We put a higher priority on a natural feel of a training model than a natural appearance. The Advanced Venipuncture Training Aid is substantially lower in cost than the anatomically correct training arms, are latex-free and has a durability of up to 7200 punctures. For more information, visit www.phlebotomy. com/TrainingAid.html.

Transfusion errors

I have been asked to monitor our lab's error rate through all phases of blood transfusion. Is there any benchmark I can refer to in order to see how our lab is doing compared to others? I am especially interested in the errors during specimen collection.

This is a worthy agenda for you to explore in your facility. You are to be commended for embarking on such a study.

Transfusing a unit of blood can involve up to ten different laboratory and healthcare professionals. Errors can occur in every step of the process. There is an interesting article in the April 2001 issue of *Laboratory Medicine* that summarizes the literature on transfusion errors.[1] It focuses on those that occur from specimen collection through administration of the unit, including preadministration verification, clerical errors, typing errors, specimen labeling errors, etc.

In summarizing the article, one third of all transfusion deaths and two thirds of all incompatible transfusions were preventable. The rate of ABO incompatible transfusion is cited as being one for every 33,000 transfusions; the fatality rate is one for every 600,000. The article also cites another study of transfusion errors that showed phlebotomist error was responsible for 11% of transfusion errors while nursing/physician ID errors totaled 43%. Blood banks were solely responsible for 25% of transfusion errors and shared responsibility for another 17%. The downside of the article is that it concerned transfusion error surveys conducted in the 1980s and '90s.

Likewise, a study published in *Transfusion* detailed the types and frequency of labeling errors that occurred when 496 patient specimens didn't match the blood bank's historical record for the patients' blood group (1.2% of all samples considered).[2] Of those that appeared properly labeled, 14 (0.035%) were found to contain another patient's blood, based on historical ABO records.

A study done on transfusion errors in New York State from 1990 to 1999 revealed a phlebotomy error rate of 13% with blood banks solely responsible for 29% of errors and a shared responsibility with 15%.[3] Interestingly, 0.5% of wristbands carried another patient's information.

References

1) Sauer D, McDonald C, Boshkov L. Errors in transfusion medicine. *Lab Med* 2001;32(4):205-207.

2) Lumadue J, Boyd J, Ness P. Adherence to a strict specimen-labeling policy decreases the incidence of erroneous blood grouping of blood bank specimens. *Transfusion* 1997;37(11–12):1169–72.

3) Linden J. Wagner K, Voytovich A, Sheehan J. Transfusion errors in New York State: an analysis of 10 years' experience. *Transfusion* 2000;40(10):1207–13.

Did You Know...

as many as 10 different healthcare workers are involved in the complex process of transfusing blood.

Underfilled tubes

I am at a cancer hospital where blood draws are frequent and so are transfusions. When we draw CBCs, chem 10s and PTs/aPTTs(INRs), does the tube need to be filled to get accurate results? We were hoping that we could use the smaller tubes (peds tubes) to limit the amount of blood taken from each patient. Any information would be helpful, especially if any research has been done on this.

Your desire to minimize the volume of blood drawn from your patients should be applauded. Using tubes of a smaller fill volume is recommended and is the best way to minimize blood volumes withdrawn.

It's well documented that if you underfill any tube, even the pediatric tubes, the results could be significantly affected. Here's why: tube manufacturers put a calculated amount of additive in their tubes to properly prepare a specimen for testing when completely filled. Underfill the tube and you tinker with this chemistry and cause "excessive anticoagulation." The only exception is the serum tubes (red tops and gold tops). They have a clot activator, but its concentration in the sample is not critical. All other tubes should be filled to the stated volume if you want to be sure the results reflect the patient's physiology.

When EDTA tubes are underfilled, for example, the excess concentration of the additive tends to shrink the red blood cells. As a result, the hematocrit and MCV will be reported out as falsely lower. The most sensitive tube to underfilling is the coagulation tube. It is imperative that it be filled to at least 90% of its stated volume.[1-3] Failure to do so can result in a dilution of the blood and a falsely elevated coagulation result. This can lead to a dangerous change in the patient's medication, and cause stroke or other complications.

References

1) CLSI. *Collection, Transport, and Processing of Blood Specimens for Testing Plasma-Based Coagulation Assays and Molecular Hemostasis Assays; Approved Guideline—Fifth Edition.* CLSI document H21-A5. Wayne, PA: Clinical and Laboratory Standards Institute; 2008.

2) Reneke J, Etzell J, Leslie S, Ng V, Gottfried E. *Coag Trans Med* 1997;109(6):754–7.

3) Castellone D. How to deliver quality results in coagulation laboratory: commonly asked questions. *Lab Med* 2004;4(35):208–213.

Did You Know...

blades that penetrate deeper than 2.0 mm
should not be used on the heels of infants.

Underfilling heparin tubes

I received a request for information today about the effect of underfilling lithium heparin tubes, and whether there was a minimum amount. We use 4 mL tubes and, because they are infrequently used, cannot really stock smaller volume tubes. Is there any literature or information about the effect of underfilling heparin tubes and increasing the proportion of anticoagulant to blood?

There isn't much in the literature on the effects of underfilling heparin tubes. As such, it's impossible to know whether or not you're getting accurate results from them.

Hypothetically, one could conduct an internal study on varying levels of underfills and compare the results of all the tests commonly performed on heparin tubes to determine the level of significant difference. The study would have to compare multiple patients, multiple analytes, and multiple ranges of each analyte. That's a lot of work and statistical analysis, but there's no other way around it. It's best to establish and enforce your fill volumes according to the manufacturer's recommendations.

Venipuncture depth

I am constantly getting the question from my students, many of whom are nurses, about how far they should insert the needle into the vein. We use inch-and-a-quarter needles. Since I am teaching people who are used to threading a long IV catheter into the vein, I tell them that, for drawing blood, they only want to penetrate the vein surface not thread the needle up the vein. Yesterday, two of the techs here at the lab took issue with that technique. What are your thoughts on the matter? How deep should I teach them to insert the needle?

The depth of the puncture is not so much a function of needle length, but depth of the vein. You go as deep or as shallow as the vein seems to be, making sure you penetrate the uppermost wall of the vein.

If your needles are 1.25 inches long and you go half the length of the needle into the arm, you're penetrating over half an inch. That sounds excessive. If a vein is a half inch beneath the skin, it's probably too deep to palpate. Rarely should a venipuncture needle have to go deeper than a quarter inch.

As you found out, those who have experience inserting IV catheters have a tendency to "thread" the needle into the vein as they would an IV. As educators, we have to reinforce diligently that inserting a needle for phlebotomy is entirely different than for starting an IV. For phlebotomy, one only needs to access the vein, then stop advancing; threading the needle further into the vein is not necessary.

Index